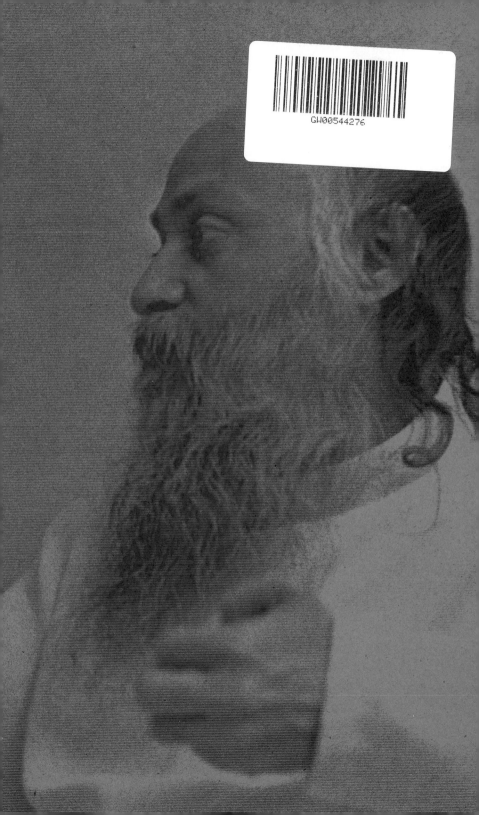
GW00544276

YOGA: THE Alpha and the Omega
VOLUME X

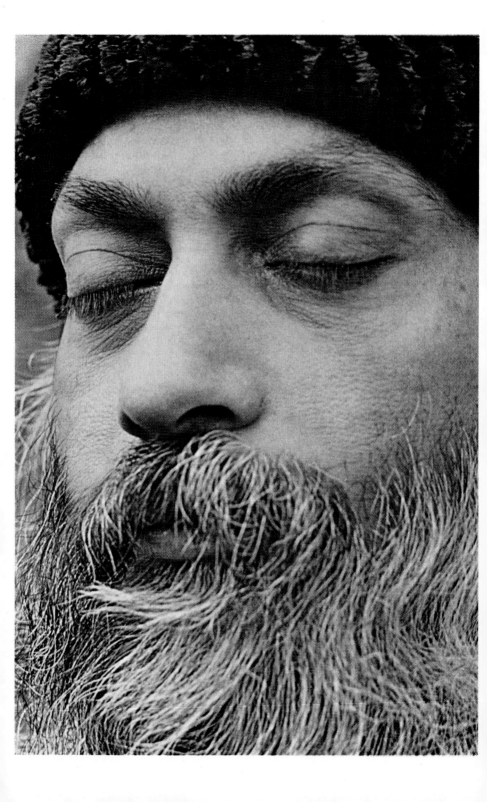

BHAGWAN SHREE RAJNEESH

Talks on the Yoga Sutras
of Patanjali

YOGA: The Alpha
and
the Omega

VOLUME X

Compilation
MA DEVA BHASHA

Editing
MA YOGA SUDHA

Design
SWAMI GOVINDDAS
SWAMI PREM DEEKSHANT
SWAMI ANAND SUBHADRA

RAJNEESH FOUNDATION

© Copyright by Rajneesh Foundation
Poona, India. All Rights Reserved

Published by Ma Yoga Laxmi
Rajneesh Foundation, Shree Rajneesh Ashram
17 Koregaon Park
Poona 411001 India

Composed by:
Beacon Typesetting, Inc.
14626 Titus St.
Panorama City, Calif. 91402

Printed by:
Arun K. Mehta
Vakil & Sons Ltd.
Vakils House
18 Ballard Estate
Bombay 400038, India

First Edition: July 1978
5,000 Copies

Printed in India

ISBN   0-88050-186-3

Photographs
SWAMI KRISHNA BHARTI
SWAMI SHIVAMURTI
MA PREM CHAMPA

Assistance
MA YOGA VIRAG
MA DEVA BHASHA

CONTENTS

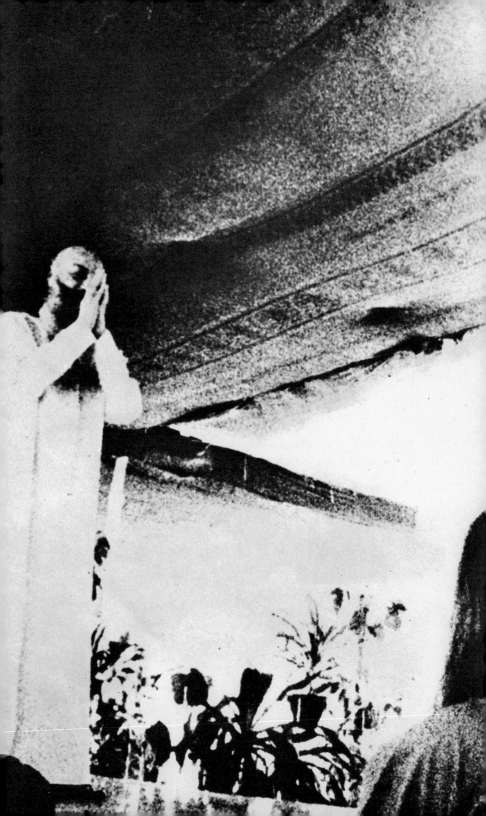

INTRODUCTION

A seeker must cross the deserts of his own being. He must plunge into the fires, strip himself and be nude before the rays of the orange sun. He must be vulnerable to the sandstorms and let the winds make him soft, supple. Like the mythical phoenix, he must rise again from his own ashes, for the ashes of defeat are but the fodder of wisdom. He may stop for refreshment at the occasional oasis, but only for moments. The journey is long, and there is such a wealth of life to be lived.

And Bhagwan has taken us through the aridity of Yoga, through the effort, the methodical, step by step going, so lovingly, so joyously that we hardly notice . . . and here we are. He has brought us to the garden, to that place from which we had never really departed.

In Bhagwan's garden there are many saplings, many flowers stretching their petals to drink in the gift of life. They roll and toss in their slumber, feeling the quickening of wakefulness to the presence of the sky. Bhagwan sits, ever so quietly, within each little growing thing, waiting for the moment when the call of life becomes audible. (That voice is such a silence.) He waits there for understanding to happen, for the quest to begin. And then he takes us.

And he has taken us. We have crossed the desert. Now, the garden . . . the omega.

ma yoga sudha

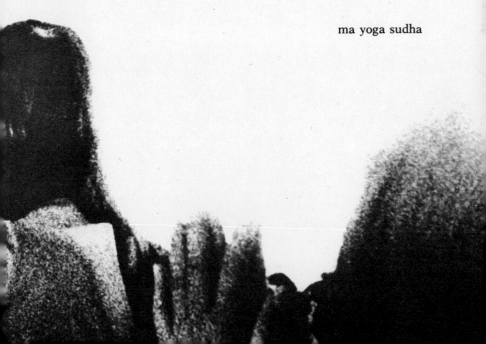

The sutras in this volume are
based on Chapter Four, *Kaivalya Pada, the*
verses 1 through 34 of the
Yoga Sutras of Patanjali ... the omega.

CHAPTER ONE
May 1, 1976

DROPPING THE
ARTIFICIAL MIND

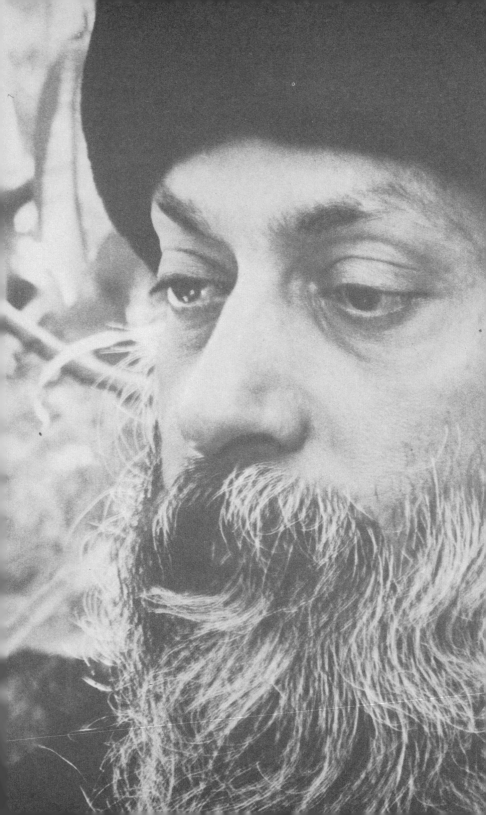

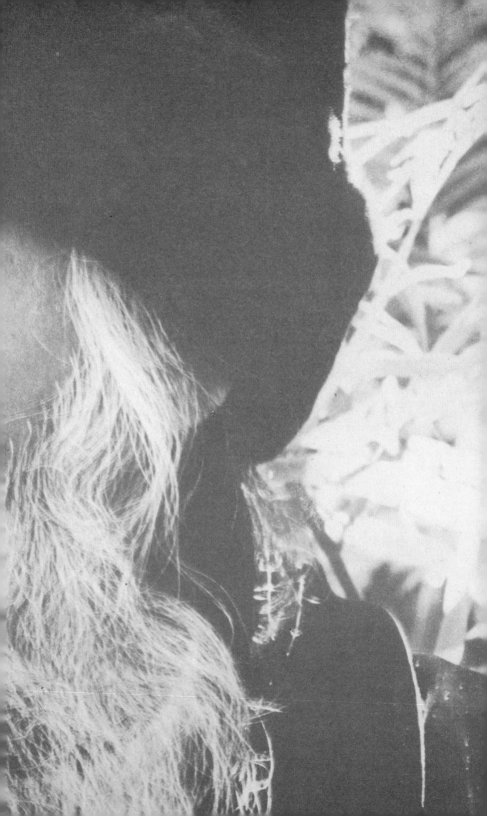

Now begins the last section of Patanjali's sutras, *Kaivalya Pada.*

1

The powers are revealed at birth, or acquired through drugs, repeating sacred words, austerities, or samadhi.

जन्मौषधिमन्त्रतपः समाधिजाः सिद्धयः ॥ १ ॥

2

The transformation from one class, species, or kind, into another, is by the overflow of natural tendencies or potentialities.

जात्यन्तरपरिणामः प्रकृत्यापूरात् ॥ २ ॥

3

The incidental cause does not stir the natural tendencies into activity; it merely removes the obstacles—like a farmer irrigating a field: he removes the obstacles, and then the water flows freely by itself.

निमित्तमप्रयोजकं प्रकृतीनां वरणभेदस्तु ततः क्षेत्रिकवत् ॥ ३ ॥

4

Artificially created minds proceed from egoism alone.

निर्माणचित्तान्यस्मितामात्रात् ॥ ४ ॥

5

Though the activities of the many artificial minds vary, the one original mind controls them all.

प्रवृत्तिभेदे प्रयोजकं चित्तमेकमनेकेषाम् ॥ ५ ॥

MAN IS ALMOST MAD—mad because he is seeking something which he has already got; mad because he's not aware of who he is; mad because he hopes, desires, and then ultimately, feels frustrated. Frustration is bound to be there because you cannot find yourself by seeking; you are already there. The seeking has to stop, the search has to drop: that is the greatest problem to be faced, encountered.

The problem is that you have something and you are seeking it. Now how can you find it? You are too occupied with seeking, and you cannot see the thing that you already have. Unless all seeking stops, you will not be able to see it. Seeking makes your mind focus somewhere in the future, and the thing that you are seeking is already here, now, this very moment. That which you are seeking is hidden in the seeker himself: the seeker is the sought. Hence, so much neurosis, so much madness.

Once your mind is focused somewhere, you have some intention. Immediately, your attention is no longer free. Intention cripples attention. If you are intently looking for something, your consciousness has narrowed down. It will exclude everything else. It will include only your desire, your hope, your dream. And to realize that which you are you need not have any intention; you need attention, just pure attention: not intending to go anywhere, unfocused consciousness, consciousness here-now, not anywhere else. This is the basic problem: the dog is chasing its own tail. It gets frustrated; it becomes almost mad because each step, and nothing comes into its hands—only failure, failure, failure.

Just the other day a *sannyasin* told me that he was now feeling frustrated. I became tremendously happy. Because when you feel frustrated, something opens within you. When you feel frustrated, if *really* frustrated, then future disappears. Future can exist only with the support of expectation, desire, intention. Future is nothing but intentionality. I became tremendously happy that one man was frustrated.

Fritz Perls, one of the very perceptive men of this century, has said that the whole work of the therapist is nothing but skillful frustration, creating frustration.

What does he mean? He means that unless you are really frustrated with your desires, hopes, expectations, you will not be thrown back to your own being. A real frustration is a great blessing. Suddenly you are, and there is nothing else. The sannyasin said, "I am feeling frustrated. It seems that nothing is happening. I have been doing all sorts of meditations, all sorts of group therapies, and nothing is happening." That's the whole point of all meditations and all group therapies: to make you aware that nothing can happen. All has happened already. In deep frustration, your energy moves back to the source. You fall upon yourself.

You will try to create new hope. That's why people go on changing their therapists, their therapies, their Masters, gurus, religions. They go on changing because they say, "Now I am feeling frustrated here; somewhere else, I will again sow new seeds of hope." Then you will be continuously missing. If you understand, the problem is: how to throw you upon yourself, how to frustrate you in your desires. Of course, it has to be very skillful.

That's what I am doing here. If you don't have any desires, first I create them. I give you hope. I say, "Yes, soon something is going to happen"—because I know that desire is there, but not full-fledged. It is there hiding in a seed form; it has to sprout, it has to flower. And when the desire flowers, those flowers are of frustration.

Then suddenly you drop the whole nonsense, the whole trip. And once you are authentically frustrated—and when I say authentically, really frustrated, I mean that now you don't start any other hope again; you simply accept it and you return back home—you will start laughing. This is what you were always seeking. And it has always been inside you, but you were too much occupied with seeking.

There is a very beautiful movie called *The King of Hearts*. The context is the First World War, and the Germans and the English are fighting over a French town. The Germans plant a time-bomb and leave the town, and the French learn about the bomb and they also leave the town.

All the people in the insane asylum come out, take over the empty town, and have a wonderful time—because nobody is left there, only the insane people of the insane asylum. Even their guards have escaped, so they are free. They come into the town and everything is empty: shops are empty, offices are empty. So they take over the town; they take over the empty town, and have a wonderful time. They all put on different clothes and enjoy themselves thoroughly. Their madness simply disappears; they are no more mad. Whatsoever they always wanted to become and could not become, now they simply became, without any effort. Somebody became the general, and somebody became the duke, and somebody the madame, and somebody else the doctor, the bishop, or whosoever he wants to become. Everything is free. They put on different clothes and enjoy themselves thoroughly. Everyone takes on some role in the town: general, duke, lady, madame, bishop, etc. One guy becomes a barber, and he pays customers because he enjoys being a barber; and he gets more customers that way.

They are all living these roles, living in the moment and enjoying it completely, utterly.

A British soldier is sent to the town to disable the bomb. He gets frustrated because he cannot find where the bomb has been put. He starts ranting and raving and shouting, "We are all going to die!" So everyone, everyone: the general, the duke, the bishop—the mad people—everyone brings lounge chairs to watch him perform. They clap and they cheer. Of course, he gets even more mad.

The next day both the Germans and the British march back into the town and all the crazy people treat it as a parade. Then the soldiers see each other, shoot and kill each other. The duke, up in a balcony, looks down disdainfully at all the bodies and says, "Now they are overacting." A young woman looks down sadly and says with puzzlement, "Funny people." The Bishop says, "These people have certainly gone mad."

You think mad people are mad . . . just look at yourself, at what you are doing. You think when a madman pretends that he is the prime minister or the president that he is mad? Then what are your presidents and prime ministers doing? In fact, they may be more mad. The madman simply enjoys the fantasy, he does not bother to make it an actuality; but the premiers, the presidents and the generals have not remained satisfied with their fantasy; they have tried to actualize it. Of course, if any madman is an Alexander or a Genghis Khan, he never kills anybody; he simply is. He does not go to prove that he really is. He's not dangerous, he's innocent. But when these so-called sane people have the idea of being an Alexander, a Genghis Khan, a Tamurlaine, then they don't remain contented with the idea. They try to actualize it. Your Adolf Hitlers are more mad, your Mao Tse Tungs are more mad than any mad people in any mad asylum.

The problem is that the whole humanity exists as if under a certain hypnosis.

It is as if you have all been hypnotized and you don't know how to get out of it. All our life-styles are insane, neurotic. They create more misery than they create happiness. They create more frustration than they create fulfillment. The whole way you live brings

you more and more, closer and closer, nearer and nearer to hell.
Heaven is just a desire; hell is almost a reality. You live in hell and
you dream about heaven. In fact, heaven is a sort of tranquilizer: it
gives you hope—but all hopes are going to be frustrated. The hope
of heaven simply creates a hell of frustration. Remember this; only
then will you be able to understand Patanjali's last chapter,
Kaivalya Pada.

What is the art of liberation? The art of liberation is nothing but
the art of de-hypnosis: how to drop this hypnotic state of mind;
how to become unconditioned; how to look at reality without any
idea creating a barrier between you and the real; how to simply see
without any desires in the eyes; how simply to be without any
motivation. That's all yoga is about. Then suddenly that which is
inside you, and has always been inside you from the very beginning, is revealed.

The first sutra:

Janmausadhi-mantra-tapah-samadhi-jah
siddhayah.

The powers are revealed at birth . . .

This is a very pregnant sutra, and I have not yet come across a
right commentary about this sutra. It is so pregnant that unless you
penetrate it to the very core, you will not be able to understand it.

The powers are revealed at birth, or acquired through
drugs, repeating sacred words, austerities, or
samadhi.

Whatsoever you are is revealed at birth without any effort. Every
child, while he is being born, knows the truth, because he has not
yet been hypnotized. He has no desires; he is still innocent, virgin,
not corrupted by any intention. His attention is pure, unfocused.
The child is naturally meditative. He is in a sort of samadhi; he's
coming out of the womb of God. His life river is yet absolutely
fresh, just from the source. He knows the truth, but he does not
know that he knows. He *knows* it, not knowing that he knows it.
The knowledge is absolutely simple. How can he know that he
knows?—because there has never been a moment of not knowing.
To feel as if you know something, you have to have some experience
of non-knowledge. Without ignorance you cannot feel knowledge.
Without darkness you cannot see stars. In the day you can't see the

stars because it is all light. In the night you see the stars because it is all dark; contrast is needed. A child is born in perfect light: he cannot feel that this is light. To feel it, he will have to pass through the experience of darkness. Then he will be able to compare and see, and know that he knows. His knowledge is not yet aware. It is innocent. It is simply there, as a matter of fact. And he is not separate from his knowledge; he is his knowledge. He has no mind, he has simple being.

What Patanjali is saying is this: what you are seeking you had known before. Not knowing it, you had known it before. Otherwise, there would be no way to seek it because we can only seek something which we have known in some way—maybe very dimly, vaguely. Maybe the awareness was not clear: it was clouded in mist; but how can you seek something which you have not known before? How can you seek God? How can you seek bliss? How can you seek truth? How can you seek the self, the supreme self? You must have tasted something of it, and that taste, the memory of that taste is still treasured somewhere within your being. You are missing something; that's why search, seeking arises.

The first experience of samadhi, the first experience of infinite power, *siddhi*, of potentiality, of being a god, is revealed at birth. But at that time, you cannot make a knowledge out of it. For that you will have to go through a dark night of the soul; you will have to go astray. For that, you will have to sin. The word 'sin' is very beautiful. It simply means going off-track, missing the right path, or missing the target, missing the goal. The Adam has to go out of the Garden of Eden. It is a necessity. Unless you miss God, you will not be able to know Him. Unless you come to a point where you don't know whether God is or is not, unless you come to a point where you are miserable, in pain and anguish, you will never be able to know what bliss is. Agony is the door to ecstasy.

Patanjali's first sutra is simply saying that whatsoever is attained by the yogi is nothing new. It is a recovery of something lost. It is a remembrance. That's why in India once somebody attains *samadhi*, we call it a rebirth; he is reborn. We call him *dwija*: twice born. One birth was unconscious, the first birth; the second birth is conscious. He has suffered, gone astray, and come back home. When Adam returns home, he is Jesus. Every Jesus has to go far away from the home; then he is Adam. When Adam starts the returning journey, he is Jesus. Adam is the first man, Jesus the last. Adam is the beginning, the alpha, and Jesus the end, the omega; and the circle is complete.

"The powers are revealed at birth. : . ." Then arises 'the world';

what Hindus call *maya*. It has been translated as illusion, magic, but the best way to translate it is as hypnosis. Then arises the hypnosis. A thousand and one hypnoses are all around: here he's being taught that he is a Hindu—now it is a hypnosis; he's being taught that he is a Christian—now it is a hypnosis. Now his mind is being conditioned and narrowed down. He's a Mohammedan—it is a hypnosis. Then he is taught that he is a man or a woman—it is a hypnosis.

Ninety per cent of your manhood or womanhood is simply hypnosis; it has nothing to do with your biology. The biological difference between man and woman is very simple, but the psychological difference is very complicated and complex. You have to teach small boys to be boys and small girls to be girls, and you bifurcate them. You create an intention: the girls are going to become beautiful women, and the boys are going to become very powerful men. The girls are going to be just confined in the home: householders, housewives, mothers; and the boys are going on a great adventure in the world: money, power, prestige, ambition. You create different intentions in them.

In different societies, different conditionings are given. There are societies which are matriarchal; the woman is predominant. Then you will see an unbelievable truth there: whenever there is a society in which the woman is predominant, the man becomes weak and woman becomes powerful. She manages all outside work and the man simply looks after the home.

But because we live in a male-dominant society, man becomes powerful and woman becomes weak and fragile. But this is a hypnosis; it is not natural. It is not so in nature. You give a certain direction, then a thousand and one sorts of hypnoses go round.

In India, if a man is born in a poor, untouchable's family, is a *shudra*, he's confined to being a shudra for his whole life. He cannot even change his business. He cannot become a *brahmin*. He's confined: a very narrow hole, a tunnel-like hole is given to him. He has to go through that; no other alternatives are available. And he will think in those terms, he will live a certain style of life. And each conditioning of the mind is self-perpetuating: it goes on creating itself more and more skillfully. Then you are given ideas about God. In Soviet Russia, you are given the idea that there is no God.

Stalin's daughter, Svetlana, has written in her memoirs that from the very beginning, of course, since she was Stalin's daughter, she was taught very strictly to be an atheist. But by and by, she started feeling, "Why? If there is no God, why is there so much propaganda against Him? What is the point? There is no point in it; if God is not there, finished. Why be worried? Why create anti-God propaganda, literature, this and that; why try to prove? The very effort shows that something seems to be there, something may be there." She became suspicious, and when Stalin died she revolted. She became a religious person, but her mind was narrowed down. She must be a very rare human being, because to be a theist in Soviet Russia is as difficult as to be an atheist in India.

These things are not taught, these things are caught—with the blood of the mother, with the milk of the mother, with the breathing of the mother. Your whole atmosphere surrounds you as a subtle conditioning. These things are not taught. Nobody is teaching you these things in particular; you catch them. The first thing a Hindu child hears when he opens his eyes and his ears here, the first thing is going to be a *mantra*, or something from the Bhagavad-Gita. He does not understand anything, but the first impact is of Sanskrit, the first impact is of some religious scripture. Then he starts growing; he sees his mother praying, the statues of gods, and flowers and incense, and he goes on crawling there, watches and sees what is happening. He can see that the mother is crying, tears are coming, and she looks so happy and so graceful. Something tremendously great is happening; he cannot know what it is, but something is happening. He is catching. Then the temple, then the priest, then the flamboyant robes, and the whole atmosphere; he goes on drinking the atmosphere. It becomes part of his being. Either from the mother's breast or from the state's breast, but these things are just caught while he is unaware. You become a Christian: by the time you become alert you are already a Christian, a Hindu, a Mohammedan, a Jaina, a Buddhist, and it is very difficult to uncondition you.

The whole effort of Patanjali is how to uncondition you, how to help you so that you can uncondition yourself. All that has been given to you has to be dropped so that again you come out of the clouds into the open sky, so that again you can come out of this small, tunnel-like existence of being a Hindu, a Mohammedan, a communist, this and that; how to find the open sky again—dimensionless. No religion, particularly no organized religion, is in favor of it. They decorate their tunnels. They force things on people, as if theirs is the only way to reach to God.

I have heard about a man, a Protestant, who died and reached to heaven. He asked Saint Peter, "First, before I settle somewhere, I

would like to have a tour. I would like to see the whole of heaven."
Saint Peter said, "Your curiosity is understandable, but one thing
you will have to remember: I will take you around, but don't talk,
be completely quiet. And walk so that no noise is made." The
Protestant was a little worried, "Why so much...?" but they
walked. Whenever he wanted to say anything, Saint Peter would
put his finger on his lips and say, "Shhh! Keep quiet." When the
tour was over he asked, "What is the matter? Why so much
quietness?" Peter said, "Everybody here believes. For example, the
Catholics believe only they are in heaven; the Protestants believe
only they are in heaven; the Hindus believe only they are; the
Mohammedans believe only they are. So they feel very much
offended if they come to know that somebody else is also there.
That is impossible for them to believe."

On the earth people live in tunnels, and in heaven also.

No organized religion can be in favor of a totally open mind.
That's why an organized religion is not a religion at all; it is a
politics.

Just the other day I received a letter from Amida. She was in
Arica. Now she has come here, so those Arican people are very
much disturbed. She has become a sannyasin, so they have written
a letter of expulsion. She is expelled. This looks like nonsense. This
seems to be politics. Now she cannot be allowed to attend their
meetings anymore, or to participate with them. In their jargon they
have said, "Now you are put in water." She is condemned. The
same goes on everywhere. Scientology does the same to people.
Once you are in scientology and you leave it, just as Amida has
been put in water, they give a notice that you are now an enemy.
An enemy!

But this is how it has always happened. Always remember,
wherever your mind is being narrowed, escape from there. It is not
religion, it is politics. It is an ego-trip.

Religion widens you.

Religion widens you so much that the whole house around you,
by and by, disappears. You are just under the sky, absolutely nude,
in total communication with existence. Nothing exists between you
and existence. This point is achieved easily, naturally, spontaneously, at the time of birth. The powers are revealed at birth—
everything is revealed at birth. It is only a question of reclaiming it.
It is a question of remembering it again. It is not going to be a
discovery, it is going to be a re-discovery.

Many people come to me and they ask, "If samadhi happens, if

enlightenment happens, how are we going to recognize it, that it is
that?" I say to them, "Don't you be worried; you will recognize it
because you know what it is. You have forgotten. Once it happens
again, suddenly, in your consciousness, the memory will arise,
surface, and immediately you will recognize."

And this can be also acquired in four ways. The first is through
drugs. Hindus have made drugs for thousands of years. In the West
the craze is very new; in India it is very ancient.

Patanjali says,
> It can be acquired through drugs, repeating sacred
> words, mantras, austerities, or samadhi.

He's in favor only of samadhi, but he's a very, very scientific man.
He has not left anything out.

Yes, it can be acquired through drugs, but that is the lowest
glimpse of it. Through chemicals, you can have a certain glimpse,
but that is almost a violence, almost a rape of God—because you
are not growing into the glimpse; rather, you are forcing the
glimpse upon yourself. You can take LSD, or marijuana, or something else: you are forcing your chemistry. If the chemistry is forced
too much, for a few moments it becomes loosened from the conditioning of the mind. From the tunnel-like style of your life it
becomes loose. You have a certain glimpse, but the glimpse is at a
very great cost. Now you will become addicted to the drug.
Whenever you need the glimpse you will have to go to the drug, and
each time you go the drug, more and more quantity of it will be
needed. And you will not be growing at all, you will not be
maturing at all. Only the drug will grow in quantity, and you will
remain the same. This is getting a glimpse of the divine at a very
great cost. It is not worth it. It is destroying yourself. It is suicidal,
but Patanjali puts it there as a possibility. Many have tried that,
and many have gone almost insane through it. It is dangerous to try
any violence on existence. One should grow naturally. At the most,
it can be like a dream, but it cannot be a reality. A person who has
been taking LSD for long remains the same person. He may talk
about new spaces that he has achieved and he will talk about
'far-out experiences', but you can see that the man has remained
the same. He has not changed. He has not attained to any grace. It
may be otherwise: he may have lost any grace that he already had
before. He has not become more happy and blissful. Yes, under the

impact of the drug he may laugh, but that laughter is also ill: it is
not arising naturally, it is not flowering naturally. And after the
impact of the drug he will be dull, he will have a hang-over; and he
will again and again seek, again and again he will seek and search
for the same glimpse. Now he will become hypnotized by the
experience of the drug. It is the lowest possibility.

The second, better than this, is of *mantra*. If you repeat a certain
mantra for a long time, that too creates subtle chemical changes in
your being. It is better than drugs, but still, that too is a subtle
drug. If you repeat, Aum, Aum, Aum, continuously, the very repetition creates sound waves in you. It is as if you go on throwing rocks
into the lake and waves arise and arise and go on spreading,
creating many patterns. The same happens when you use a mantra,
the continuous repetition of any word. It has nothing to do with
Aum, Ram, Ave Maria or Allah; it has nothing to do with them. You
can say,."Blah, blah, blah"; that will do. But you have to repeat
the same, the same sound with the same tone, in a rhythm. It goes on
falling on the same center again and again, and creating ripples,
vibrations, pulsations. They move inside your being and spread out.
They create circles of energy. It is better than drugs, but it is
still of the same quality.

That's why Krishnamurti goes on saying that mantra is a drug.
It is a drug, and he is not saying anything new; Patanjali says the
same. It is better than the drug: you don't need any injection, you
are not dependent on any outside agency. You are not dependent on
the drug-pusher because he may not be giving you the right thing.
He may be handing you something bogus. You need not depend on
anybody. It is more independent than drugs. You can repeat your
mantra inside you, and it is more in tune with the society. The
society will not object that you repeat: Aum, Aum, Aum, but if you
take LSD the society will object. Chanting is better, more respectable, but still a drug. It is through sound that the chemistry of
your body is changed.

Now, much experimentation is going on with sound, music,
chanting. It certainly changes chemistry. A plant grows faster if it
is surrounded by music—by a certain music of course—classical or
Indian; not by modern Western music. Otherwise, the growth stops,
or, the plant goes crazy With subtle vibrations, with great rhythm
and harmony, the plant grows faster. The growth is almost doubled
and the flowers come bigger, more colorful; they live longer and
they have more fragrance. Now these are scientific truths. If a plant
is affected so much by sounds, much more will happen to human

beings. And if you can create an inner sound, a continuous vibration, it will change your physiology, your chemistry—your mind, your body—but it is still an outside help. It is still an effort: you are doing something. And by doing you are creating a state which has to be maintained. It is not naturally spontaneous. If you don't maintain it for a few days, it will disappear. So, that too is not a growth.

Once a Sufi visited me. For thirty years he had been doing a Sufi mantra, and had done it really sincerely. He was full of vibrations—very alive, very happy, almost ecstatic the whole day, as if in samadhi . . . drunk. His disciples brought him to me. He stayed with me for three days. I told him, "Do one thing: for thirty years you have been doing a certain chanting; stop for three days." He said, "Why?" I said, "Just to know whether it has happened to you yet or not. If you go on chanting you will never know. You may be creating this drunkenness by chanting continuously. You drop it for three days and just see." He became a little afraid, but he understood the point.

Because unless something becomes so natural that you need not do it, you have not attained to it.

Just within three days, everything disappeared; just within three days! A thirty-year effort, and after the third day the man started crying and he said, "What have you done? You have destroyed my whole *sadhana!*" I said, "I have not destroyed anything; you can start again. But now remember, if you repeat for thirty lives even, you will not attain. This is not the way. After thirty years, you cannot go for a three-day holiday? That seems to be a bondage, and it has not yet become spontaneous. It has not yet become part of you; you have not grown. These three days have revealed to you that for thirty years the whole effort has been in the wrong direction. Now it is up to you. If you want to continue, continue. But remember, now don't forget that any day it can disappear; it is a dream that you are holding through continuous chanting. It is a certain vibration that you are holding, but it is not arising there. It is cultivated, nurtured; it is not yet your nature."

The third way is by austerities, by changing your way of life, not hankering for comfort, convenience: for food, for sleep, for sex; dropping all that the mind naturally desires and doing just the opposite. That is still a little higher than mantras. If the mind says go to sleep, the man of austerities says, "No, I'm not going to sleep. I am not going to be a slave to you. When I would like to go to sleep, I will go; otherwise not." The mind says, "You are feeling hungry, now go and beg"; the man of austerities says, "No!" The man of austerities says no continuously to his mind. That is what austerity is: saying no to the mind. Of course, if you continuously say no to the mind, the conditioning becomes loosened. Then the mind is no longer powerful over you, then you are released a little. But that no has to be said again continuously. Even if you listen to the mind for one day, again the whole power of mind will return to dominate and possess you. So just a moment's going astray, and all is lost.

The man of austerities is doing better; he is doing something more permanent than the man of chanting—because when you chant, your life-style remains unchanged. Just inside, you feel good: a certain well-being. That's why Maharishi Mahesh Yogi's Transcendental Meditation has so much appeal in the West, because he does not ask you to change your life-style. He says, "Whatsoever, wherever you are, it's okay." He does not want you to make a disciplined life; simply repeat the mantra, twenty minutes in the morning and twenty minutes in the evening, and that will do. Of course, it will give you better sleep, a better appetite. You will be more calm and quiet. In situations where anger was easy, it will not be so easy. But you have to continue the chanting every day. It will give you a certain inner bath in sound waves. It will give you a little cleansing, but it is not going to help you grow. Austerities help more because your life starts changing.

If you decide not to do a certain thing, the mind will insist that you do it. If you go on denying the mind, your whole life pattern changes. But, that too is forced. People who are in austerities too much lose grace, become a little ugly. Constant struggle and fight, and constant repression and saying no creates a very deep rift in their beings. They may have more permanent glimpses than the man of chanting or the man who is addicted to drugs. They will have more permanent results than Timothy Leary and Mahesh Yogi, but still, it is not a spontaneous flowering. It is still not Zen, not real Yoga, not Tantra.

... or samadhi.

Then comes the fourth which Patanjali has been trying to explain to you. Through *samyama*, through samadhi, everything has to be attained. Whatsoever he has been teaching up to now is through samyama, samadhi—bringing your awareness to it. The man of drugs works through the chemistry; the man of austerities works through the physiology; the man of chanting works through the sound-structure of his being, but they are all partial. His totality is not yet touched by them. And they all will create a sort of lopsidedness. One part will grow too big, and other parts will lag behind, and he will become ugly.

Samadhi is the growth of the total.

And the growth has to be natural, spontaneous, not forced. The growth has to be through awareness; not through chemistry, not through physics, not through sound. The growth has to be through awareness, witnessing: that's what samadhi is. Samadhi will bring you to the same point when you were born. Suddenly, it will reveal your being to you, who you are.

Now, a few things about samadhi will have to be understood.

One: it is not a goal to be achieved, it is not a desire to be achieved. It is not an expectation, it is not a hope, it is not in the future; it is here-now. That's why the only condition for samadhi is desirelessness—not even the desire for samadhi.

If you desire samadhi, you are continuously eroding samadhi yourself. The nature of desire has to be understood, and in that understanding it drops by itself, on its own accord. That's why I say that when your hopes are frustrated, you are in a beautiful space; use it. That is the moment when you can enter into samadhi more easily.

Blessed are those who are hopeless: let it be added to Jesus' other beatitudes.

He says, "Blessed are the meek, because they shall inherit the earth." I say to you: blessed are the hopeless, because they will inherit the whole.

Try to see how hope is destroying you. With hope arises fear. Fear is the other side of the same coin. Whenever you hope you also become afraid. You become afraid of whether you are going to fulfil your hope or not. Hope never comes alone; it keeps company with fear. Then, between fear and hope you are spread out. Hope is in the future and fear is also in the future, and you start swinging between hope and fear. Sometimes you feel, "Yes, it is going to be fulfilled"; and sometimes you feel, "No, it seems impossible," and fear arises. Between fear and hope, you lose your being.

Let me tell you one very famous old Indian story.

A fool was sent to buy flour and salt. He took a dish in which to carry his purchases. He was told not to mix the two ingredients, but to keep them separate. After the shop-keeper had filled the dish with flour, the fool, thinking of the instructions, inverted the dish asking that salt be poured on the upturned bottom. Therewith the flour was lost, but he had the salt. He brought it to his boss who enquired, "But where is the flour?" The fool turned the dish over to find it, so the salt was gone too.

Between hope and fear, your whole being is lost.

That's how you have become so disintegrated, split, schizophrenic. Just see the point of it: if you don't have any hope, you will not be creating any fear—because fear cannot come without hope. Hope is a step of fear in you. Hope creates the door for the fear to enter. If you don't have any hope then there is no point in fear. And when there is no hope and no fear, you cannot move away from yourself. You are simply that which you are. You are here-now. This moment becomes intensely alive.

The second sutra:

Jaty-antara-parinamah prakrty-apurat.

The transformation from one class, species, or kind into another is by the overflow of natural tendencies or potentialities.

Very significant. . . .

If you are a man of austerities you will not be overflowing. You will have repressed your energies. Afraid of sex, afraid of anger, afraid of love, afraid of this and that, you will have repressed all your energies; you will not be in an overflow. And Patanjali says that only through overflow is there transformation. It is one of the most basic laws of life.

Have you watched that when you are feeling low in energy, suddenly love disappears? When you are feeling low in energy, creativity disappears. You cannot paint, you cannot write a poem. If you write, your poetry will not walk; dancing is far away. It will not even walk; it may, at the most, limp. It will not be much of a poem. If you paint when you are low-energy, your painting will be ill. It will not be healthy. It cannot be because it is your painting and you are feeling low in energy. In fact, the painting is you spread on the canvas. It will be gloomy, sad, dying.

I have heard about one great painter who had asked one of his friends, a doctor, to come and see his painting. The doctor watched, looked from this side and that. The friend, the painter, was very happy at how much he was appreciating. Then he finally asked, because he saw that the doctor was looking puzzled—not even puzzled, but worried. The friend said, "What is the matter? What do you think of this painting?" He said, "Appendicitis." He had made a portrait of somebody and the doctor was looking everywhere, because the face was so pale and the body looked in such agony that he felt it must be appendicitis. Later on, it was found that the painter had the appendicitis, he was suffering from it.

You spread yourself in your poetry, in your painting, in your sculpture. Whatsoever you do, it is you; it has to be so.

Flowers come into the trees only when they are overflowing; the energy's too much. They can afford it. When a tree has not much energy, it will not flower because it has not even energy enough for the leaves. It has not even energy enough for the roots—how can it afford? Flowers will be almost a luxury. When you are hungry, you don't bother to buy paintings for your house. When you don't have clothes, you think of clothes; you don't think of having a beautiful garden. These are luxuries. When energy is overflowing, then only is the celebration, the transformation. When you are overflowing with energy you want to sing, you want to dance, you want to share.

The transformation from one class, species or kind into another is by the overflow . . .

Ordinarily, as man is, he is so blocked and there are so many problems repressed that the energy never comes to a point where it can overflow and just be shared with others. And your *sahasrar*, which is your flowering, the lotus in the crown of your head, will not flower unless energy is overflowing, unless it is overflowing so much so that it goes on rising higher and higher. The level goes on rising higher and higher; it reaches to the second center, the third center, the fourth center, and whatsoever center is touched by the overflowing energy opens, flowers. The seventh *chakra* is the flower of humanity: *sahasrar*. *Sahasrar dul kamal:* the one-thousand-petalled lotus that will flower only when you are in an overflow.

Never repress and never create blocks in your being. Never become too solid. Don't get frozen. Flow. Let your energy remain always streaming. That's the whole purpose of yoga methods: that your blocks are broken. The yoga postures are nothing but just a methodology to break the blocks that you create inside your body.

Now, something exactly like it has happened in the West. It is Rolfing, founded by Ida Rolf. Because in the West the mind is more technological, people don't want to do their own thing. They want it to be done by somebody else; hence Rolfing. The Rolfer will do the work. He will give you deep massage, and he will try to melt your blocks. The musculature that has become hardened will be relaxed.

The same can be done with yoga, and more easily, because you are your own master. You can feel your inner being more rightly, accurately. You can feel where your blocks are. If you close your eyes and sit silently every day, you can feel where your body is feeling uncomfortable, where your body is feeling tense. Then there are yoga *asanas* for that particular body part to relax. Those asanas will help to dissolve the musculature which has become hardened and will allow the energy to move. But one thing is certain: that a repressed person never flowers.

A repressed person remains with dammed energy, pent-up energy. And if you don't channelize your energy in right directions, your energy can become destructive and suicidal to you. For example: if your energy is not moving towards love, it will become anger. It will go sour, bitter. Whenever you see an angry person remember, somehow his energy has missed love. Somehow, he has gone astray; hence, he is angry. He is not angry at you, he is simply angry; you may be just an excuse. He is anger. The energy is blocked and life is feeling almost meaningless, without any significance; he is in a rage.

There is a very famous poem of Dylan Thomas. His father died, and on that night he wrote this poem. In this poem come the lines,

> Rage, rage against the dying
> of the light:
> Do not go gently into that
> good night!

He is saying to his father "Fight with death; rage against it. Don't surrender, don't just let go. Give a good fight even if you are defeated, but don't go without a fight."

If love is not fulfilled, one becomes angry. If life is not fulfilled, one becomes angry at death. A man whose life is a fulfillment will not rage against death, he will welcome. And he will not say that it is dark night; he will say, "So beautiful, so restful." The dark is restful. It is almost warm, like mother's womb. One is moving again into the greater womb of God. Why rage? Those who have flowered, surrender. Those who are frustrated cannot surrender. Out of their frustrations they create more hopes, and each hope brings more frustrations—and the vicious circle goes on and on, ad nauseam.

If you want not to be frustrated, drop hope—then there will be no frustration. And if you want really to grow, never repress. Enjoy energy. Life is an energy phenomenon. Enjoy energy—dance, sing, swim, run—let energy stream all over you, let energy spread all over you. Let it be a flow. Once you are in a flow, flowering becomes very easy.

> *The incidental cause does not stir the natural*
> *tendencies into activity; it merely removes the*
> *obstacles—like a farmer irrigating a field: he removes*
> *the obstacles, and then the water flows freely by*
> *itself.*

Patanjali is saying that, in fact, if you don't have blocks everything will be attained naturally. It is not a question of creating anything; the question is only of removing the blocking. It is as if a spring is there, and a rock is blocking its way. It is streaming behind it, but cannot remove the rock. The spring, the water, has not to be created, it is already there; you simply remove the rock and it bursts forth. It is like a fountain: you just remove the rock and it bursts forth, it flowers. The child has it naturally; you have to attain it by understanding. And, you have to drop all the blocks that the society has enforced upon you.

The society is against sex: it has created a block, just near the sex center. Whenever sex arises you feel restless, you feel guilty, you feel afraid. You shrink; you don't stream, you don't flow. The society is against anger: it has created a block there. So anger comes, but you cannot move into it totally. You will have to drop all these blocks.

That's why I insist for dynamic methods: they will melt your blocks. If you are angry, scream, yell. There is no need to yell and scream at anybody; just a pillow will do. Beat the pillow, jump on it, kill the pillow—there is no need to kill anybody. Just the idea that you are killing the pillow is enough. Just getting into the rage, into the anger, is enough; the block is broken. If you want to kill somebody, or if you want to be angry at somebody, you can never be totally in it—impossible—because the other is going to be hurt, wounded, and you are a human being: you have compassion and love also. So one withholds.

Beat the pillow. Have a good knife and kill the pillow. When the pillow is dead, bury the body and be finished with it. Suddenly, you will feel that something has broken inside you. A rock has been

removed. Yell, jump, jog. If sex arises, help it to arise. Forget all
that the society has taught you. Enjoy the very feeling of sensuality
arising in you. Cooperate with it. Don't shrink and don't resist it;
cooperate with it. Soon you will see that the sensuality is transforming. When the pool is full, it starts overflowing. Sensuality
overflowing becomes sensitivity. People who repress their sex become insensitive, dull. They don't have life. They become wooden.

The incidental cause does not stir the natural
tendencies into activity; it merely removes the
obstacles.

The whole effort of yoga is to remove the obstacles, *via negativa*.
Nothing is really to be done because you have everything; it is just
not flowing. A few rocks have been put on the path. You have been
distracted. It is just like a farmer irrigating a field. Have you seen a
farmer irrigating a field? Water is flowing in one channel; he
removes a little earth and the water starts moving into that path.
When that part is irrigated he puts a little earth back on the gate;
the water stops flowing on that path. Then he opens the channel
somewhere else; the water starts flowing there. Water is there; it
needs channelization. Energy you have, you are; it simply needs
channelization so it reaches to the *sahasrar*, to the highest peak, the
climax of your being.

Artificially created minds proceed from egoism alone.

And we all have artificial minds. That's what I call the hypnosis
that society has done to you.
We have a group in the ashram, and I have been thinking about
it. It is called 'Hypnotherapy', but I would like to call it 'de-
Hypnotherapy'—because the basic effort is to de-hypnotize you, or
unhypnotize you, uncondition you.
All minds are artificially created minds: *Nirmana cittany
asmita-matrat*. Artificially created minds proceed from egoism
alone: I am a Hindu, I am a Mohammedan, I am black, I am white,
I am this, that—they are all artificial minds. The original face, the
original mind, uncreated by man, has to be known and realized.
I have heard: A little colored boy accidentally spilled a tin of
white paint over himself. When he arrived home, his father gave
him a good hiding and told him to go straight to bed. Sobbing his

way out of the room he said, "I have only been white for twenty minutes, and I hate you blacks already!"

Even a twenty-minute-old child has started accumulating the artificial mind. Even a twenty-minute-old child looks at his mother with more love than towards anybody else, because he has learned one trick. The conditioning has started: she is food, and survival depends on food. So howsoever ugly the mother, the mother always looks beautiful. It is survival, and the child has started learning diplomacy. He will not smile so much at the father. He does not know who this man is. He will learn it later on. By and by, he will see that this man is important. Of course, he is not seen very much in the home, but important. Rarely, on Sundays he is there, but even the mother depends on him, even the mother smiles at him. Then the child also smiles at the father. He is learning the artificial mind. He's creating relationships, arranging his survival, creating a situation—diplomacy, politics—but this artificial mind which is a help in survival in the beginning, becomes the greatest problem in the end.

When you have survived and you have used the artificial mind, then it hangs around you like a rock around your neck. It becomes the ego. It has to be learned; nothing can be done about it. Every child will have to move into the artificial mind. But when you become alert and aware, and when you start thinking and meditating about life, then it is time to, by and by, drop it. And drop the ego, because the ego is nothing but the artificial mind. The center of the artificial mind is the ego. And every artificial mind can be continued only if you go on enhancing your ego.

Hindus will say that they have the greatest religion in the world, that they are the most religious people in the world. In fact, if they were really religious they would not utter such nonsense, because a religious mind is humble, simple. This is ego. Then every country has its own ego. The Russian, the Chinese, the American, the German, the English—everybody has his own ego, and every country goes on feeling that, "We are the superb, the chosen." Every country finds ways and means to feel enhanced, as with every race, every group, and every man and woman.

I have heard: The elephant looked down and saw a little, very tiny mouse standing by its foot. "Dear me," said the elephant, "you are very tiny." "Yes," agreed the mouse, "I have not been very well lately." Even a mouse has his own ego?—he has been ill, that's why.

The artificial mind lives through ego, so if you start dropping your ego, the artificial mind will start disintegrating. Or, if you drop your artificial mind, the ego will start disintegrating. And if you really want to get rid of this rock, start both ways together. Never enhance the ego in any way. The ways are very subtle.

Remember that the original mind is egoless. It does not know the 'I', because 'I' is a shrinking. The original mind is infinite, like the sky.

And one problem arises continuously as far as ego is concerned. In the beginning you try to befool others about yourself, but, by and by, you are befooled yourself. When you start convincing others that you are somebody in particular, you become convinced yourself.

There was a strict rule in the mental asylum: no pets. The warder heard poor Harry talking to a dog called Rover, and marched into his padded cell. There was Harry, leading a tube of toothpaste around on a piece of string. "What is that?" asked the warder. Harry looked at him in surprise. "Surely any fool can see it is just a tube of toothpaste on a piece of string!" he said. Satisfied, the warder left. Just as he closed the door behind him, Harry breathed a sigh of relief. "Good boy, Rover. We sure fooled him that time."

The more you try to befool others, to prove that you are some-body in particular, exceptional, extraordinary, this and that—all neurotic ideas—the more you succeed in proving it to others, the more you will only succeed in befooling yourself. Look at the whole nonsense of it.

Nobody is extraordinary, or, everybody is extraordinary. Nobody is special, or, everybody is special. But there is no point in proving anything either way—there is no need.

Artificially created minds proceed from egoism alone, so if you want to come to the original mind—which is the whole effort of Yoga, Tantra, Zen—then you will have to drop the artificial mind; the mind that has been created by the society and given to you; the mind that has been created from the outside and enforced on you. By and by, drop it. The more you see, the more you will be able to drop. Whenever you start feeling attached to the artificial mind: whenever you say, "I am a Hindu, and I am an Indian; or, I am English, I am British"; or this and that, just catch yourself red-handed. Deep inside, slap your face, and say "What nonsense!" By and by, don't be defined by society. Then you will find the indefina-ble; your real, authentic being.

*Though the activities of the many artificial minds
vary, the one original mind controls them all.*

So whatsoever your artificial mind, in fact, in reality, the original mind hiding behind it controls them all. Find the controller. Try to find who you originally are before the society corrupted you, contaminated you, before the society entered, planned you, and destroyed your wildness. In Zen they call it: finding the original face which you had before you were born, and which you will have when you will again die; the original face, untouched by society. That's your nature, your soul, your being.

Finding the original face, you will be reborn, you will become a *dwij*, twice-born. You will become really a brahmin, one who knows. Then again everything will be revealed to you as it was revealed at the time of birth, because you will be born again. But this time, there is going to be a great difference: you will be alert. The first time you missed; you will not miss this time. The first time it happened naturally; this time it will happen with your alertness, your awareness. You will be conscious of it. You will see yourself reborn again, being born again, arising out of the past, out of the clouds and confusion—thoughts, prejudices, egos, minds, conditionings—arising out of them, virgin, pure. Then you will again see the *power* that you are, the being that you are.

So first, it happens at birth; second it happens at samadhi; in between, it can be managed by three methods—drugs, chanting, austerities—but those·three methods are ways of deceiving, cheating. And you cannot cheat upon God, you can cheat yourself; remember that.

CHAPTER TWO
May 2, 1976

ALONENESS IS THE LAST
ACHIEVEMENT

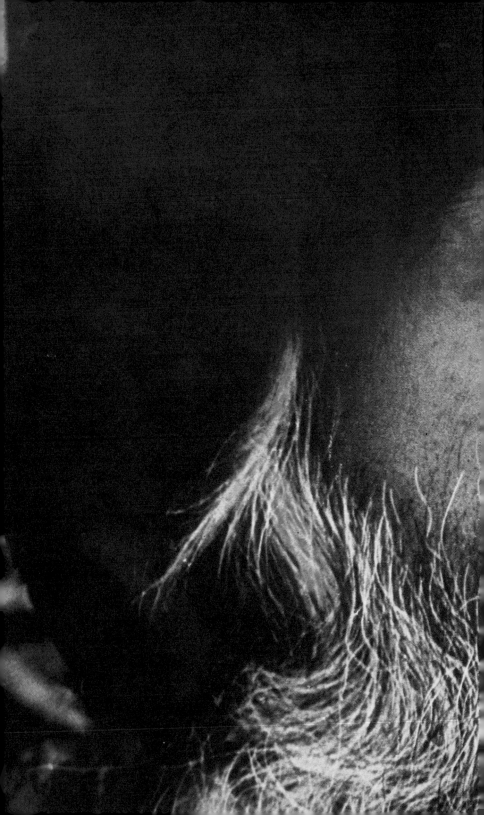

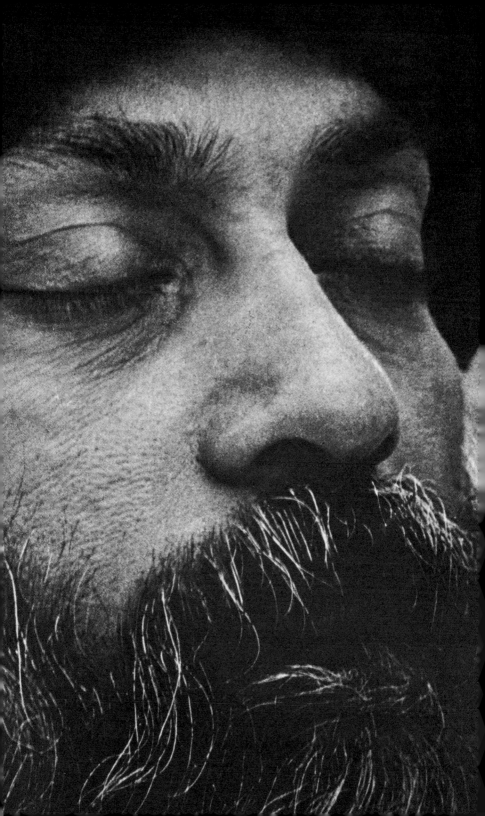

The first question:

Does a disciple steal something from his Master?

EVERYTHING!
Because the truth cannot be taught, it has to be learned.
The Master can only tempt you, make you more and more
thirsty for it; but he cannot deliver it to you—it is not a
thing. He cannot simply transfer it in your name—it is not a
heritage. You will have to steal it. You will have to work hard in the
dark night of the soul. You will have to find ways how to steal it.
The Master only tempts you; he simply provokes you. He shows
that something is there, a treasure, and now you have to work hard.
In fact, he will create all sorts of obstacles so that you cannot reach
to the treasure very easily. Because if you reach to the treasure very
easily, you will not have grown; you will lose that treasure again. It
will be a treasure in the hands of a child. The key will be lost, the
treasure will be lost.

So not only do you have to steal, but the Master has to work in
such a way that you become able to steal only when you are ready.
He has to create many obstacles. He goes on hiding the treasure. He
will allow you only when you are ready. Just your greed or your
desire is not enough, but your readiness, your preparedness; you
have to earn it. And it is like stealing because the effort has to be
made in the dark, and the effort has to be made very silently. And
there are a thousand and one obstacles on the path, temptations to
go away, temptations to get distracted. The help of the Master is
really to make you more skillful, to give you the knack of how to
feel whether the treasure exists here or not.

Living with the Master, surrounded by his climate, slowly,
slowly, a certain awareness arises in you. Your eyes become clear
and you can see where the treasure is. And then, you work hard for
it. The Master gives you a glimpse of the far-away peak of the
Himalayas—snow-covered, shining in the sun—but it is far away
and you will have to travel. It is going to be hard, it is going to be
uphill. There is every possibility that you may get lost. There is
every possibility that you may miss the goal, you may go astray.
The closer you come to the peak, the possibility of missing becomes

bigger and bigger, greater and greater—because the closer you come to the peak, the less you can see the peak. You have to move just by your own alertness. From far away you can see the peak; it is difficult to lose the direction. But when you have reached the mountains and you are moving upward, you cannot see the peak. You have simply to grope in darkness, so it is more like stealing. The Master is not going to give to you easily. It can be allowed very easily—the door can be opened right now—but you will not be able to see any treasure there because your eyes are not trained yet. And even if, just on trust, you believe that this is very, very valuable, you will lose your trust again and again. Unless *you* feel and know that this is valuable, it is not going to be kept for long; you will throw it anywhere.

I have heard about a poor man, a beggar, who was coming with his donkey on the road. The donkey had a beautiful diamond just dangling on his neck. The beggar had found it somewhere and thought it looked beautiful, so he had made a little ornament for the donkey, a necklace. One jeweller saw it. He reached to the poor man and asked, "How much will you take for this stone?" The poor man said, "Eight *annas* will do." The jeweller became greedy. He said, "Eight *annas?*—for just this small stone? I can give you four *annas.*" But the poor man said, "For four *annas* why take it away from the donkey? Then I'm not going to sell." The jeweller said that the beggar would sell, so he went a little far away. He would come back to persuade. But by that time, another jeweller saw it. He was ready to give one thousand *rupees,* so the poor man sold immediately because the other was not even ready to give eight *annas.* And this jeweller looked almost mad; one thousand rupees he offered! The first jeweller came back but the diamond was gone. He said to the poor man, "You are a fool! You have sold it just for one thousand *rupees;* it was worth almost one million rupees!" The beggar laughed, "I may be a fool—I am—but what about you? I did not know that it was a diamond, and you knew it and you would not take it even for eight *annas.*"

You can get the diamond; it will be taken away from you. You cannot keep it for long. It will be stolen unless you yourself understand how valuable it is. So you have to grow.

The work of the Master is very paradoxical. The paradox is: he provokes you, he invites you, and goes on hiding the treasure. He has to do both simultaneously: he has to tempt you, seduce you, and yet, he is not to allow you an easy approach. Between these two very paradoxical efforts: provoking, continuously provoking. . . .

I go on speaking every day; this is nothing but temptation, an invitation. But I will hide it to the last unless you have become capable of stealing. I am not going to give it; it cannot be given. You can only steal it. But you will become, by and by, a master thief. The temptation will make you. What will you do? I will tempt you and nothing will be given to you. What will you do?—you will start thinking of how to steal it.

Nothing happens before its right time; truth, at least, never happens before its right time. And if I try to give it to you, it will never reach you in the first place. Even if it reaches, you will lose it again. And . . . it will not be an act of compassion on my part if I give it to you. My compassion has to be hard. My compassion has to be so hard that you go on crying for it and I go on hiding it. On the one hand, I tempt you; on the other hand, I hide it. Once tempted, you will become, by and by, crazier and crazier. You will find ways; you have to find ways. Because only through finding, searching, seeking ways, inventing, innovating, enquiring new paths, getting out of the old patterns, finding new patterns, new disciplines, will you grow, will you become rich. In fact, the moment you have grown, suddenly the truth is there within you. One just has to recognize it, but that recognition comes the hard way. You will have to stake everything that you have: that is the meaning of stealing. It is not a business: it is not a bargain. It is like stealing.

Think of the thief: he stakes everything for something which is not known, which he doesn't know whether it is really there or not. He stakes his property, he stakes his family, he stakes his own life. If he misses and something goes wrong, he may be in prison forever. He's a gambler; very courageous. He's not a businessman. He stakes everything for something which may be there or may not be there. The businessman has a dictum: he says, "Never lose your half bread in the hand for a whole bread in the future, in imagination. Never lose that which you have for that which you don't have." That is the dictum of the businessman, the businessman's mind.

The thief follows another dictum totally: he says, "Put everything that you have at stake for something that you don't have." For his dream, he stakes the real. It is just a 'perhaps'. He risks all his securities for something very insecure. That's where courage is.

So rather than being a businessman, be a thief, be a gambler. Because the unknown can be found only when you are ready to drop the known. When the known ceases, the unknown enters into your being. When all security is lost, only then do you give way for the unknown to enter in you.

The second question:

> *Cannot one enjoy life alone? Because I am not so aware, that*
> *moving into water without getting wet, or going through fire*
> *without getting burnt can be possible for me. Cannot one enjoy*
> *life alone?*

At least the questioner cannot enjoy, because one who can enjoy
will never ask the question.

The very question shows that it will be impossible for you to
enjoy being alone. Your aloneness will deteriorate and become
loneliness. Your aloneness will not be a fullness; your aloneness
will be loneliness—empty.

Yes, out of fear you can settle in it. Out of the fear of getting wet
in the water, out of the fear of getting caught in the fire; out of fear,
you may settle. Many have settled. Go to the monasteries; look into
the old ashrams: many have settled just out of fear.

Relationship is a fire; it burns. It is difficult. It is almost impossible to live with someone. It is a constant struggle. Many have
escaped, but they are cowards. They are not grown-ups; their effort
is childish. Yes, they will live a more convenient life, that's true.
When the other is not there, of course, everything goes easily. You
live alone—with whom to get angry?—with whom to get jealous?—
with whom to fight? But your life will lose all taste. You will become tasteless; you will not have any salt.

Many escape from life just because life is too much, and they
don't find themselves capable of coping with it. I will not suggest
that; I am not an escapist. I will tell you to fight your way through
life, because that is the only way to become more aware and alert;
to become so balanced that nobody can unbalance you; to become
so tranquil that the presence of the other never becomes a distraction. The other can insult you but you are not irritated. The other
can create a situation in which, ordinarily, you would have gone
mad, but you don't go. You use the situation as a stepping-stone for
a higher consciousness.

Life has to be used as a situation, as an opportunity to become
more conscious, more crystallized, more centered and rooted. If you
escape, it will be as if a seed escapes from the soil and hides in a
cave where there is no soil, only stones. The seed will be safe. In
soil, the seed has to die, disappear. When the seed disappears, the
plant sprouts. Then dangers start. For the seed there was no
danger: no animal would have eaten it, and no child would have
broken it. Now the beautiful green sprout, and the whole world

seems to be against it: the winds come and they try to uproot it, clouds come, and thunders come, and the small seed is fighting alone against the whole world. There are children and there are animals and there are gardeners, and millions of problems to be faced. The seed was living comfortably, there was no problem: no wind, no soil, no animals—nothing was a problem. It was closed completely into itself; the seed was protected, secure.

So you can go to a cave in the Himalayas: you will become a seed. You won't sprout. Those winds are not against you; they give you an opportunity, they give you challenge, they give you an opportunity to get deeply rooted. They tell you to stand your ground and give a good fight. That makes you strong.

You see, one eucalyptus tree is here. Just to protect it, Mukta placed a bamboo by the side when the tree was small. Now it has gone so long, but it cannot stand on its own. The bamboos are still there and now it seems impossible. Once you remove the bamboos, the whole tree will fall down. The protection will have proved to be dangerous. Now the tree has become accustomed to protection. It has not grown in strength, it has remained childish.

Challenges are growth opportunities, and there is no greater challenge in life than love. If you love someone, you are in a tremendous turmoil. Love is not all roses as your poets say; they are all fools. They may have dreamed about love but they have never known it. It is not all roses. It is more thorny than you can imagine. Roses are rare, here and there; thorns are millions. But when out of a million thorns a rose arises, it has a beauty of its own. Love is the greatest danger in life. That's why I insist that if you really want to grow, accept the greatest danger and move into it.

People have tried to find many ways of avoiding it. Some have left the world. Why are you so afraid of the world? The fear of the world is really fear of love, because when others are there, the possibility is there that you may fall in love with someone. There are so many beautiful souls around, so many attractions; you may get caught somewhere. Danger . . . escape! A few have escaped to the monasteries, a few have escaped in other ways. A few have escaped into marriages. That too is an escape. The monastery is an escape, and marriage is also an escape—to avoid love.

One never knows what will be the outcome of a love affair. It is always on the rocks. It is never convenient, it is never comfortable. It may bring you moments of joy, but it brings hell also. It is painful growth, but all growth is painful. One never grows without pain. Pain is part, an essential part. If you avoid the pain you also avoid the growth.

Many have settled somewhere. A few have settled in ambition, have become politicians. They are not worried about love. They say they have great things to do in the world. They are worried about power: they use power as an escape. A few are buried in their monasteries, a few are buried in their families: marriage, children, this and that, but I rarely come across a man who has faced the challenge of love, the greatest storm there is. But one who has faced it, grows. He comes out of it one day, clean, pure, mature.

So you ask, "Cannot one enjoy life alone?"

You can be happy alone, but you cannot enjoy. You can be happy, in a way, because there will be no disturbance, no turmoil, no conflict. Your happiness will be more like peace, less like enjoyment. It will not have any ecstasy in it. Joy is very ecstatic; joy is very much like dance. Happiness is like the singing you do in your bathroom—the bathroom singing—it is very lukewarm; you can do it alone. You always do it in your bathroom because you are alone. But singing and dancing with other people, getting completely possessed by it, is joy. Joy is a shared phenomenon; happiness is a non-shared phenomenon.

People who are miserly always look for happiness, not for joy— because joy needs sharing. You cannot be joyful alone. A certain atmosphere is needed, a certain climate is needed: a certain whirlwind of people, persons, consciousness, is needed. Alone you can be happy, at the most.

And remember, happiness is not a very happy thing.

Joy is really moving high. Joy is the climax, like peaks; happiness is a plain ground: one moves comfortably with no fear of any fall anywhere—no valley around, no danger. You can walk with your eyes closed. You know the path. You have been moving on that path, this way and that. You can move completely unconsciously.

Joy needs consciousness. Have you ever moved into the mountains and just by the side, a great valley is yawning? You become alert. That is one of the beauties of mountaineering. It is not really the joy in the mountain; the joy is in moving in danger, constant danger. Always there is death around; the valley is waiting to swallow you at any moment. Once you lose your footing, you are gone forever. Because of that danger one becomes very sharply aware, like a sword. That awareness gives joy.

When you are moving with people, in relationship, you are always in danger. Life becomes sharp. Then you have a tone; then

your energy is not just rusting, it is flowing. Look at the people who
have lived too long in the caves or in the monasteries: you will see
that a certain rust has settled on their faces. They will not look
alive. They will be dull almost to the point of being stupid. That's
why monks have not created anything beautiful in the world.
Nothing has come out of them. They are wastages; they are not
fertile soil. They proved impotent.

All escape makes you more of a coward, impotent. And the more
you escape, the more you want to escape. All escape is suicidal.

Then what do I mean? Am I saying to you, never be alone? No,
not at all. But I am saying, never be lonely. Aloneness comes out of
the richness that you have learned through relationships, out of
many relationships, of many dimensions, many qualities: being
with a mother, being with a father, being with a friend, being with
a brother, sister, being with a wife, being with a beloved, lover,
with friends, with enemies. 'Being with' is the world. And one has
to be in as many relationships as possible; then you expand. Each
relationship contributes something to your inner enrichment. The
more you spread into people, the more you expand. You have a
bigger soul, and you have a richer soul. Otherwise, you become
impoverished.

Now psychoanalysts have been working hard on children who
have not received their first and basic relationship: the relationship
between the child and the mother. They shrink. These children are
never normal. Somehow, the first urge to expand has not happened.
The relationship between a child and the mother is the first entry
into the world.

You enter into the world with your mother's love. You enter into
the world because you relate with your mother, and you learn how
to relate. The warmth that flows between the child and the mother
is the first exchange of energies. It is tremendously sexual, because
all energy is sexual. The child smiling, the mother smiling, a
tremendous energy is being exchanged. The mother cuddling the
child, hugging the child, kissing the child; a great energy is being
given to the child, and the child is getting ready to respond. Sooner
or later, the day will come when the child will hug and kiss the
mother. Now he's ripe—not only ready to take, but ready to give
also. That is his first learning. Then he will move with brothers and
sisters and father and uncles, and the circle will become bigger and
bigger and bigger: in school, and in college, and in the university,
and then in the universe—one goes on.

The more and more you relate, the more and more you are. The being is discovered through being related. Each relationship is a mirror. It shows a fragment of your being to you. It reflects something about yourself. When you have grown so much and expanded to the infinity, then the last relationship is with God.

That is the last relationship.

If you escape from relationship, as these so-called religious people do. . . . They are doing something very absurd. They will not be able to relate with God because they have not learned how to relate. They have not learned how to move in relationship. And remember, to relate with God is the greatest, the most dangerous relationship there is.

Just the other day I was reading a memoir of a Christian, a very beautiful person who had lived in Soviet Russia's jails for many years. For three years continuously he was in an underground cell, thirty feet into the earth. For three years continuously he never saw any sunlight, any flower, any butterfly, any moon. He didn't see any human face, except the guard. For three years it was maddening: no book to read, nothing to do. He was not even aware of whether it was day or night, whether the sun had arisen outside in the world or not. There was no newspaper, no news of what was happening in the world, nothing. He was completely unrelated. He started doing one thing—tremendously beautiful: he started talking to God. What to do? What else to do? For three years he talked to God and, by and by, he started giving sermons. God was the only audience. He would stand and he would give a sermon. But those sermons are really beautiful. Now, out of the jail, he has collected those sermons, and he has put them as he had given them to God. He says, "Don't be offended," because many times he becomes angry with God. One has to become. What nonsense: for three years! He quotes from scriptures and says to God, "Look at what you have said. In the Bible you say that a man should never be alone. What about me! Have you forgotten all about your scripture and your message that you gave through Jesus? Where are you? Have you changed your rules? A man should never be alone?—then why have you forced me for three years to be alone?" And he says, "Remember, at the last day of judgement I am not going to be the only culprit, you are also going to be the culprit. Not only will you tell about my sins, I am also going to tell about your sins. Remember! Don't forget it! It is not going to be one way."

Really, those sermons are beautiful, those talks with God. He remained sane because of these talks. He came out perfectly sane, saner really than when he had gone in—more sane. Such a beauti-

ful relationship ... and the God was absolutely silent. It irritates.
You go on talking; he never says yes, no—nothing.

Just think—you go on speaking and your wife keeps quiet. She
goes on working in the kitchen. You are going crazy and you are
shouting and yelling, and she goes on silently doing her things.
How will you feel? The same happens in relationship with God.
One has to learn it in life, then you can relate with God. To relate
with God is to relate with the whole. Of course, the whole is silent,
and great skill is needed in relating—only then. After you have
related with God, and you have become merged with Him, then
aloneness arises.

Aloneness is the last achievement.

That's what Patanjali calls kaivalya: absolute aloneness. It is not
in the beginning; it is in the end. That is why we are reading the
last chapter. The chapter is about aloneness, Kaivalya Pada. It is
the whole effort of the yogi through many lives to reach to aloneness. It is not so cheap as you think: that you just leave the house
and you go into a cave, and you are alone. Then there is no need for
Patanjali's Yoga Sutras. A simple sutra will do: go to the railway
station, purchase a ticket, and go to the Himalayas—finished. Who
is preventing you? Who can prevent you? How can you be pre-
vented?

But that way, life would be too cheap, would not be of worth.
One has to learn it. Aloneness is the flowering of all your relationships. You have gathered the fragrance out of all your relationships:
good and bad, beautiful and ugly; you go on gathering fragrance.
Then, a flame arises in you. That aloneness has to be the goal. What
you call aloneness right now is not aloneness; it is going just to be
loneliness. To be solitary is not to be in solitude. To be solitary is
ugly, ill, sad. To be in solitude has a tremendous beauty in it; it is
an achievement.

"... because I am not so aware, that moving into water without
getting wet, or going through fire without getting burnt can be
possible for me."

Then how are you going to become aware? Move more and more.
By escaping you will never become aware. All these situations are
needed to make you aware. If you cannot become aware in the
world, you cannot become aware out of the world. Otherwise, why
has the world been given to you; why are you in the world?—to
learn awareness.

When so many people are criss-crossing your path, so many
energies criss-crossing all around you, and it is a puzzle to solve,

awareness will arise out of it. Yes, one day you will be able to walk in water and the water will not touch your feet; but before that happens, you will have to walk in many rivers and many oceans of life. Yes, one day you will be capable of walking into fire and the fire will not burn you, but that has to be learned through many fires, and many burnings. Only out of experience is one freed. Truth liberates; experience gives you truth. Never decide for the life of no experience. Always decide for more experience. Howsoever hard and difficult, but always choose the life of experience. One day, you will transcend, but one transcends only by knowing it.

The third question:

In reply to my question, you said the other day to live and enjoy life totally. But what is life then?—to go in sex, to make money, to fulfil worldly desires, and all that? If so, then one has to depend on others, and the worldly things which are sure to become a bondage in the long run. And also, will it not make the search of the seeker very, very long?

Yes, life is all that you can imagine and desire. Sex is included, money is included; everything that the human mind can desire is included. But you live in a sort of hang-over. Even in the formulation of a question, your condemnations are absolutely clear, emphatically clear.

You say, "In reply to my question, you said the other day to live and enjoy life totally. But what is life then—to go in sex, to make money, to fulfil worldly desires, and all that?" The condemnation is clear. You seem to know the answer before you have asked the question. Your learning is absolutely clear: cut sex, cut love, cut money, cut people. Then what sort of life would be left there?

This has to be understood: the word 'life' has no meaning in it if you go on cutting everything. And everything can be condemned. Enjoying food is life; anybody can condemn it: "What nonsense! Just chewing food and swallowing it inside? Can this be life? Then breathing—just taking air in, throwing it out, taking it in, throwing it out—what boredom! And for what? Then getting up early in the morning and going to sleep in the evening, and going to the office and to the shop, and a thousand and one miseries. Is this life? Then making love to a woman? Just two dirty bodies! Kissing a woman— nothing but an exchange of saliva and millions of germs. Think of

germs: it is not even hygienic; certainly it is irreligious. It is
also unhygienic."

So what is life? Take everything out of the context of the whole,
and it looks meaningless, absurd. That's how religious people have
been condemning life through the ages. You give them anything,
and they will be able to condemn it. They say, "What is the body?
Just in a bag of skin there are millions of dirty things. Just open the
bag and see." And you will find that then they are right. But have
you asked the other question? These people must have been expecting something which they have not found. Were you expecting gold
inside the bag of skin, or diamonds inside the bag of skin? Then
would things have been better? Ask the other question: what were
you expecting? You cannot find a better and more beautiful body
than you have, and you go on looking at the dirt inside. You don't
look at the beautiful work it continues.

The whole body continues to work for seventy, eighty, or even a
hundred years with such smooth efficiency, with such silence. Look
at the throbbing energy in the body, the pulsation of energy. But
there are people who can always find something wrong. Whatsoever it is, they can find something wrong. You show them a rose
and they will take it off the plant and will say, "What is it? It will
be dead within a few hours. Yes, it will wither, so all beauty is
lost." You show them a beautiful rainbow, and they will say that it
is illusory: "You go there and you will not find anything. It simply
appears to be." These are the great condemnors, the poisoners of
life. They have poisoned everything, and you have listened to them
too much. Now you find that it has become almost impossible for
you to enjoy life. But you never think that this incapacity to enjoy
life is created by your so-called religious teachers. They have
poisoned your being. Even when you are kissing a woman, they go
on inside telling you, "What are you doing? This is nonsense. There
is nothing in it." Even while you are eating they go on saying,
"What are you doing? There is nothing in it." Those condemnors
have done a great work.

And this is one of the basic problems: that to appreciate is
difficult, and to condemn is easy. To appreciate is very difficult
because you have to prove something positively. Only then can you
appreciate. Heinrich Heine, one great German poet, writes in his
memoirs: "One day I was standing with the great philosopher,
Hegel, and it was a beautiful cool night—dark, silent—and the
whole sky was beautifully full of stars." Of course, the poet started
appreciating it, and he said, "What beauty; what tremendous

beauty!" And he added, "I always think that if a man only looks at the earth and never looks at the sky, he may become an atheist. But a man who looks at the sky, how can he become an atheist?—impossible!" But, by and by, he became a little uneasy because Hegel was completely silent; he had not uttered a word. He asked Hegel, "What do you think, sir?" And Hegel said, "I can't see any beauty or anything. These stars you are talking about?—they are nothing but a leprosy of the sky." Leprosy. . . !

Condemnation is so easy. That's why condemnors are so articulate. People have not talked in favor of life because it is difficult to say anything positive about life—it is too much for words. Condemnors have been very articulate: they have been condemning and negating, and they have created a certain mind in you which goes on working from the inside and goes on poisoning your life. Now you ask me, "What is life—to go in sex? to make money? to fulfil worldly desires, and all that?" And what is wrong in worldly desires? In fact, all desires are worldly. Have you come across any desire which is not worldly? What do you desire God for?—and you will find the whole world hidden there in your desire. What do you desire heaven for?—and you will find the whole world hidden there. Those who know say that desire is the world. They don't say 'worldly desires'. Buddha has never said 'worldly desires'. He says, "Desire is the world"; *desire as such*. The desire for samadhi, the desire for enlightenment, is also worldly. To desire is to be in the world; not to desire is to be out of the world.

So don't condemn the worldly desire; try to understand it, because all desires are worldly. This is the fear: that if you condemn the worldly desires, you will start creating new desires for yourself which you will call unworldly, or other-worldly. You will say, "I am not an ordinary man. I am not after money. What is it, after all? You die—you cannot take the money with you. I'm seeking, searching for some eternal wealth." So are you unworldly, or more worldly? People who are satisfied with the wealth of this world—which is momentary, and death will take it away—they are worldly. And you are searching for some wealth which is permanent, which is forever and ever; and you are unworldly? You seem to be more cunning and clever.

People are making love to ordinary human beings—they are worldly. And what are you desiring? And look in the Koran, look in the Bible, look in the Hindu scriptures: what are you desiring in heaven?—beautiful damsels made of gold, never aging, remaining always young. They are always at the age of sixteen—never fifteen, never seventeen—something miraculous. When the scriptures were written, then too they were at the age of sixteen. Now the scriptures have become very ancient, but those girls continue to be at the age of sixteen. What are you desiring?

In Mohammedan countries homosexuality has been prevalent, so even that is provided for in heaven. You will not only have beautiful girls, you will have beautiful boys available. And in this world alcohol is condemned, and there, in the Mohammedan heaven, there are springs of wine. Springs! You need not go to the pub, you can just swim in them, drown in them. And you call these people unworldly? In fact, they are nothing but very worldly people who have become so frustrated with this world that now they live in fantasy. They have a fantasy world; they call it paradise, heaven, or something else.

All desires are worldly, and when I say that, I am not condemning them—I am simply stating a fact: to desire is to be worldly. Nothing is wrong in it. God has given you an opportunity to understand what desire is. In understanding desire, in the very understanding of it, the desire disappears. Because desire is in the future, desire is somewhere else, and you are here-now. You want to be here-now; and the reality is here-now, the existence is happening here-now, everything is converging on here-now, and with your desire you are somewhere else so you go on missing. You remain always hungry because that which can satisfy you is showering here, and you are somewhere else.

Now is the only reality, and here is the only existence. Desire takes you away.

Try to understand desire: how it goes on deceiving you, how it goes on taking you away on further trips, and you go on missing. So whenever you remember, come back, come back home.

There is no need to fight with the desire, because if you fight with the desire you will create another desire. Only one desire can fight with another desire. Understanding is not a fight with desire. In the light of understanding desire disappears, as darkness disappears when you kindle a lamp.

So don't call these worldly desires; don't be a condemnor. Try to understand.

"If so, then one has to depend on others, and the worldly things which are sure to become bondage in the long run." But what is wrong in depending on others? The ego does not want to depend on anybody. The ego wants to be independent. But you are dependent. You are not separate from existence, you are part of it. Everything is joined together. We exist together, in a togetherness. Existence is a togetherness, so how can you become independent? Will you not breathe then? Will you not eat food? If you will eat food, you will have to depend on the trees, on the plants. They are supplying food to you. Will you not drink water?—then you will have to depend on rivers. And will you not need the sun?—then you will die. How can you become independent?

'Independent' is a wrong word, as wrong as the word 'dependent'. Independence and dependence are both wrong. The real thing is 'interdependent'. We are all together, interdependent. Even the king is dependent on his slave, as much as the slave is dependent on the king. It is an interdependence.

It happened in the life of Caliphas Haru-an-Rasid. He was sitting with his court joker, Bollul, and he said, "Bollul, I'm the most independent man in the world. I'm a monarch with infinite power, and whatsoever I want I can do. The whole world obeys me. Can you find anything which is not under my order?"

Bollul kept silent, then he said, "Sir, this one fly is disturbing me very much. Can you order her not to disturb me?"

Haru-an-Rasid said, "You are a fool. How can I order the fly? And she will not listen to me."

Bollul said, "Have you forgotten sir, what you were saying: that the whole world follows your orders?—and even this fly just in front of you is sitting on my head. I am trying to avoid it, and it goes on landing again and again on my nose; and I have seen it landing on your nose also, sir! And you cannot order this small fly?—and the whole world follows your order? You think again."

The world is an interdependence.

Haru-an-Rasid and flies are all interdependent, and Bollul is wiser than Haru-an-Rasid. In fact, because he is very wise is why he's thought of as a fool. Or, maybe it is because of his wisdom that he calls himself a fool—because to exist in this world of fools you should not declare that you are a wise man. Otherwise, they will kill you. This Bollul seems to be wiser than Socrates and Jesus. They committed one mistake: they declared that they were wise. That created trouble. All the fools gathered together and they said, "We cannot tolerate you." You cannot crucify a Bollul. Maybe he is wiser than Jesus and Socrates. He says, "I am a fool, sir"; but see his insight.

Once Haru-an-Rasid wrote a poem. Now, everybody appreciated it; everybody had to appreciate. It was just nonsense. And when he

asked Bollul before the court, he said, "This is just nonsense. Even
a fool like me, sir, will not write this." Of course, Haru-an-Rasid
was very angry. Bollul was thrown into imprisonment, and he was
beaten and forced to starve. After seven days, again he was brought
to the court. Haru-an-Rasid had written another poem, and had
improved much upon the first. And the whole court said, "Rah,
rah!" Again Bollul was asked. He looked at the poem, he listened,
and immediately stood up and started to leave. The King said,
"Where are you going?" He said, "To the prison. Again I am going.
I will not give you the trouble of sending me. What is the point?"
He was really a wise man.

This is the irony: that many times the wise man has to appear as
a fool. Remember, the effort to be independent is very foolish. And
it is not possible; it is impossible. Then you will become more and
more frustrated, because always you will find that you are again
dependent, again dependent. Wherever you go you will remain
dependent, because you cannot go out of the net of existence. We
are like the knots of a net—energies go on passing through us. When
many energies pass through a point, that point becomes an indi-
vidual, that's all. Draw a line on paper, then draw another line
across it; where these two lines cross, individuality arises. Where
life and death cross, you are there—just a crossing point.

To understand it, is all. Then you are neither dependent nor are
you independent; both are absurdities. Then you are simply interdependent, and you accept.

"If so, then one has to depend on others, and the worldly things
which are sure to become bondage in the long run." Who has told
you that they are sure to become bondage in the long run? Either
you know or you don't know. If you know, then there is no point in
asking me; you will not get into that bondage. If you don't know
and you have simply heard it from others, this is not going to help
you. You will be in trouble.

You will always be half-hearted because it is not your understanding, and only your understanding can liberate you.

Let me tell you a few anecdotes.

A man and his wife made a pact that whichever one of them died
first would come back and tell the other one what it was like on the
other side. "There is just one thing, though," said the husband. "If
you die first, I want you to promise me that you will come back
during the daytime." He was afraid, half-hearted.

If you have believed others—because others say that if you move
in the world, you will be in bondage—then wherever you move, you

will be in bondage because it is not your understanding. Understanding frees you. And remember, the bondage does not happen in the long run; it happens immediately.

The moment you desire, that very moment, the bondage has happened. It is of desire, and the desire has arisen around you; you are already imprisoned. If you have the insight, you will immediately see that every desire brings an imprisonment with it, and not in the long run. The long run . . . the very idea of long run arises because others say so. This is not your own experience. And always remember to accept your own experience; nothing else is of worth.

It happened in a court: "I notice," said the judge to the tramp in the dock, "that in addition to stealing this money, you also took a lot of very valuable jewellery." "Yes, Your Honor," remarked the tramp cheerfully. "You see, me mother taught me from childhood that money alone does not bring happiness."

Teachings from others are not going to help. You will change their whole meaning according to you. It will happen unconsciously, not consciously. You read the Dhammapada: you don't read Buddha's words, you read your own interpretations. You read Patanjali's Yoga Sutras: you don't read Patanjali, you read yourself through Patanjali. So if you are ignorant, you will find something in Patanjali which helps your ignorance. If you are greedy, you will find something in Patanjali which helps your greed. If you are greedy, you may become greedy for kaivalya, for liberation, nirvana. If you are an egoist, you will find something which helps your egoism. You will start becoming a great independent being. How can you depend? . . . such a great man. How can you depend on anybody else?—you have to be independent. You will always find yourself whatsoever you read, whatsoever you listen to, unless you start understanding your own life.

"And also, will it not make the search of the seeker very, very long?"—this is greed. Why be afraid? Why be too concerned with the result? I am saying continuously, repeatedly, to be here-now; don't think of the tomorrow. And you are not thinking only of tomorrow, you are thinking of future lives.

"Will not the search become too long, very, very long?" Why be afraid of it? Infinity is available. There is no shortage of time. You can move very, very slowly; there is no hurry. The hurry is because of the greed. So whenever people become very greedy, they become very hurried and go on finding more ways to gain more speed. They are continuously on the run because they think that life is running out. These greedy people say, "Time is money." Time is money? Money is very limited; time is unlimited. Time is not money; time is eternity. It has always been there and will be there, and you have been always here and you will always be here.

So drop greed, and don't be bothered about the result. Sometimes it happens that because of your impatience, you miss many things. If you are listening to me with greed, with greedy eyes, then you will not be listening to me. You will inside be continuously talking: "Yes, this is good; this I will try. This I will do. This seems that it will bring me to the goal very soon." You have missed me, what I was saying, and in listening to what I was saying, the goal was hidden there.

One doctor used to come here; now he is transferred. He used to take continuous notes. I asked him, "What do you go on doing?" He said, "Later, at home, with ease, I read it. And then, later on, whenever I need, I can read it again." But I told him, "You go on missing me. You hear one thing—you write—in that time I have said something which you have missed. Again you write something, again you have missed. And whatsoever you collect are fragments, and you will not be able to join them together. You will fill the gaps with your own greed, your own understandings, your own prejudices, and then the whole thing will be destroyed."

The goal is here.

You have just to be silent, patient, alert. Live life totally. The goal is hidden in life itself. It is God who has come to you as life in millions of ways. When a woman smiles at you, remember, it is God smiling at you in the form of a woman. When a flower opens its petals, look, watch—God has opened his heart in the form of a flower. When a bird starts singing, listen to it—God has come to sing a song for you. This whole life is divine, holy. You are always on holy ground. Wherever you look, it is God that you look at; whatsoever you do, it is to God that you are doing it; whatsoever you are, you are an offering to the God. That's what I mean: live life, enjoy life, because it is God. And He comes to you and you are not enjoying Him. He comes to you and you are not welcoming Him. He comes to you and finds you sad, aloof, uninterested, dull.

Dance, because each moment He is coming in infinite ways, in millions of ways, from all directions. When I say live life in totality, I mean, live life as if it is God. And *everything* is included. When I say life, everything is included. Sex is included, love is included, anger is included; everything is included. Don't be a coward. Be brave and accept life in its totality, in its total intensity.

The last question:

Can one be intimate with your soul without being your disciple?

It is as if you ask, "Can one be intimate with you without being intimate with you?"

What is a disciple?—a disciple is just an attitude, a readiness to be intimate. A disciple is just a receptivity, a readiness to accept, welcome. A disciple is a gesture: if you give to me, I will not reject it. But you are fogged with words. You have lost all insight into love, intimacy. If you are not a disciple you will not be intimate from your side. From my side, I am intimate to all, whether they are my disciples or not. I am unconditionally intimate.

But if you are not a disciple from your side you are closed, so my intimacy alone won't work. It will not get connected with you. You will remain an outsider. Somehow, you will remain in a defending mood. Of course, you will choose whatsoever you like, and you will reject whatsoever you don't like. A disciple is one who says, "Bhagwan, I accept you totally. Now I will not be a chooser with you"—that's all. "Now I drop my mind; you become my mind. I will listen to you and not to my mind. If there is any conflict, I will go with you and not with my mind"—that's all. "If a decision has to be taken, then you will be closer to me than my own mind"— that's all.

One who is not a disciple stands on the border and he says, "Whatsoever I like, or whatsoever I feel convinced of, I will choose; and whatsoever I don't like and don't feel convinced of I will not choose." Whatsoever you like will make your mind more and more strengthened; whatsoever you don't like will not allow your mind any transformation. You will become more knowledgeable. You will learn many things from me, but you will not learn me. So it is up to you.

It is not a question, for me, to make you a disciple; it is up to you. When more is available, you decide for less—so far, so good.

Let me tell you one anecdote.

A doctor had two patients from different ends of town, both chronic insomniacs. To help get some sleep, he gave them some sleeping pills. One got green pills and the other, red ones. One day, both got into conversation about their sleeplessness, and at the end of the talk, one man felt so annoyed that he rushed to his doctor and said, "How is it that when I take my pills, I go to sleep and dream I am a docker unloading a dirty tramp steamer in Liverpool, getting covered in oil and filth, while Mr. Brown takes his pills and dreams that he is lying on a beach in Bermuda, surrounded by half-dressed beautiful girls, all caressing him and kissing him and giving him a good time?" The doctor shrugged and said, "Be reasonable, now. You are on the National Health, and Mr. Brown is a private patient."

So, only that much can I say to you: be reasonable!

CHAPTER THREE
May 3, 1976

RETURNING TO
THE ORIGINAL MIND

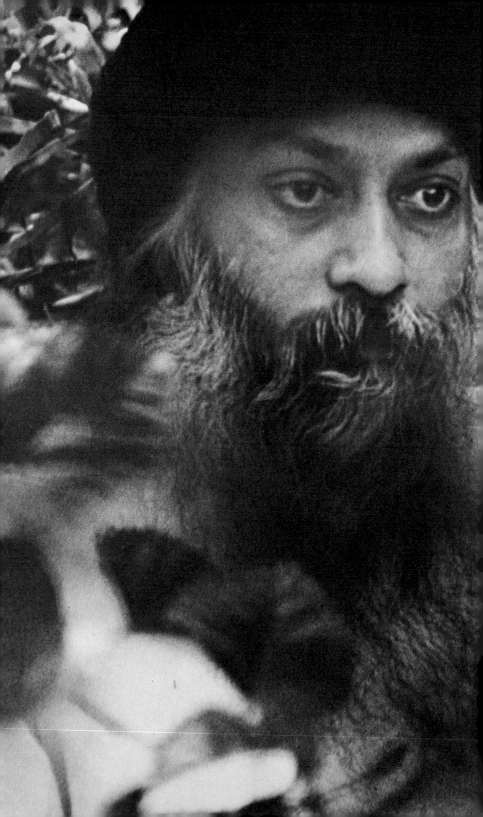

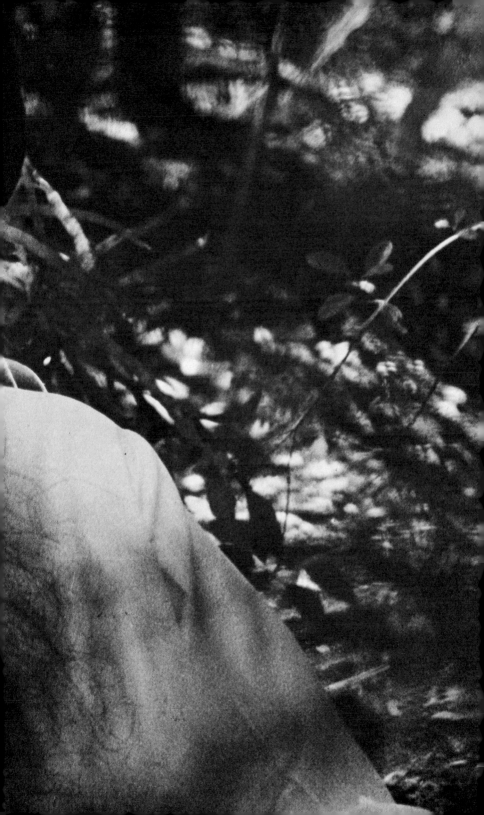

6

Only the original mind which is born of meditation is free from desires.

तत्र ध्यानजमनाशयम् ॥ ६ ॥

7

The yogi's karmas are neither pure nor impure, but all others are three-fold: pure, impure and mixed.

कर्माशुक्लाकृष्णं योगिनस्त्रिविधमितरेषाम् ॥ ७ ॥

8

Desires arise from these three-fold karmas when circumstances are favorable for their fulfillment.

ततस्तद्विपाकानुगुणानामेवाभिव्यक्तिर्वासनानाम् ॥ ८ ॥

9

Because memories and impressions retain the same form, the relationship of cause and effect continues, even though separated by class, locality, and time.

जातिदेशकालव्यवहितानामप्यानन्तर्यं स्मृतिसंस्कारयोरेकरूपत्वात् ॥ ९ ॥

10

And there is no beginning to this process, as the desire to live is eternal.

तासामनादित्वं चाशिषो नित्यत्वात् ॥ १० ॥

Tatra dhyanajam anasayam.

Only the original mind which is born of meditation is free from desires: this is one of the most significant sutras.

FIRST, WHAT IS THE ORIGINAL MIND?—because the original mind is the very goal of all yogas. The East has been searching continuously the path to the original mind. The original mind is that mind which you had before you were born, not in this life, but before you entered the world of desires; before you were confined to thoughts, desires, instincts, body, mind; that original space, uncontaminated by anything; that original sky, unclouded—that's the original mind.

On that original mind, layers and layers of minds are there. A man is like an onion; you go on peeling it. You peel one layer, another layer is there; you peel that layer, another layer comes up. You don't have one mind, you have layers and layers of many minds. Because in each life you have cultivated a certain mind, then in another life another mind, and so on and so forth. And the original mind is lost completely behind these minds, these layers upon layers. But if you go on peeling the onion, a moment comes when only emptiness is left in your hands. The onion has disappeared.

When minds disappear, then arises the original mind. In fact, to call it a mind is not good, but there is no other way to express it. It is a no-mind. The original mind is a no-mind. When all the minds that you have, have been dissolved, dropped, the original appears with its pristine purity, with its virginity. This original mind you have already. You may have forgotten. You may be lost in the jungle of your mind's conditionings, but deep down, hidden behind all these layers you still live in your original mind, and in rare moments, you penetrate to it. In deep sleep, when even dreams have stopped, in dreamless sleep, you have a dip into the original mind. That's why in the morning you feel so fresh. But if there has been a continuity of dreams the whole night, then you feel tired. You feel more tired than you were feeling when you went to bed. You could not have a dip into your inner Ganges, into your stream of pure consciousness. You could not move into it, you could not bathe in it. In the morning you feel tired, worried, tense, confused, divided. You don't have the harmony that comes out of deep sleep. But it is not coming out of deep sleep; deep sleep is just a passage to the original mind. That's why Patanjali says that samadhi is like deep sleep with only one difference: in samadhi, you move into the same original mind that you move into in sleep, but you move fully aware; in deep sleep, you slip into it unawares, not knowing where you are going, not knowing what path you are following. That's your only contact left with the original mind.

Doctors and physicians know well that whenever somebody is suffering from a disease, if he cannot sleep well, then there is no way to cure him. Sleep is therapeutic. In fact, the first thing for the patient is: how to help him move into deep sleep, deep rest. That rest cures because the patient becomes again connected with the original mind, and the original mind is a healing source. It is your source of life-energy, love. All that you have is coming from the oceanic world of your original mind.

Of course, when it has to pass so many layers of mind, it is contaminated, polluted. Your inner ecology is no longer original. It has been filled up, stuffed with many dead things. Your minds are nothing but your dead experience.

A person who wants to move into the original mind alert, aware, has to learn how to unlearn, how to unlearn the experience, how to die to the past continuously, how not to cling to the past. One moment you have lived—finished—be finished with it. Let there be no continuity with it; become discontinuous. It no longer belongs to you. It is finished and finished forever. Let it be a full point, and you get out of it as a snake moves out of the old skin and does not even look back. Just a moment before, that skin was part of his body; now, no more. Move out of the past continuously so that you can remain in the present. If you can remain in the present, you cannot go out of your original mind. The original mind knows no past and no future.

What you call the mind is nothing but past and future, past and future—a swing between past and future—and your mind never stops here-now. That's the meaning of meditation: to get out of the past, not create the future, and remain with the reality that is available here-now. Remain with it. Suddenly, you will see there is no mind between you and the reality, between you and that which is, because mind cannot exist in the present. You cannot think about it, because the moment you think about anything it is already the past, or, it is not yet present. Thinking needs time. Hence, the sutra, that only through meditation does one come to the original mind.

Meditation is not thinking; it is dropping of thinking.

I have heard: An old tramp was on the dole and he was asked what he did all day long. "Well," he said, "sometimes I sits and thinks, and other times I just sits."

That 'just sits' is exactly the meaning of meditation. In Japan they call meditation zazen. 'Zazen' means: just sitting and doing nothing, just being and doing nothing; in a state of suspended mentation. And clouds open, and you can see the space, the sky. Once you know how to move in that space, it is available always. You can go on working and whenever you want, you can have a dip inside. It becomes so easy, as if you move inside the house and outside the house. Once you know the door, there is no problem in it. You don't even think about it. When it is feeling too hot, you move inside the house, into the coolness and the shelter. When it is feeling too cold and you are freezing, you move out of the house into the hot sun. You become fluid between the inner and the outer.

The mind is blocking the path to the inner. Whenever you go within yourself, again and again you find some layer of mind: some thought fragment, some desire, some planning, some dream, something of the future or something of the past. And remember, future is nothing but a projection of the past. Future is again asking for the past in a slightly modified way, a little better. In the past you had happinesses and unhappinesses, pleasures and pains, thorns and flowers. Your future is nothing but flowers, thorns deducted, pains dropped—just pleasures and pleasures and pleasures. You go on sorting out your past, and whatsoever you feel was good and beautiful, you project it into the future.

Once you know how to get out of the past, future automatically disappears. There being no past inside, there cannot be any future. Past produces the future. Past is the mother of the future, the womb. When there is no past and no future, then what is, is. Then what is, is! Then suddenly, you are in eternity.

This is what the original mind is: with no flicker of thought, no cloud in sight, no dust around you. Just pure space.

Tatra dhyanajam anasayam.

Only the original mind is free from desires . . . because the original mind is free from the past, free from experiences. When you are free from experiences, how can you desire? Desire cannot exist without the past. Just think: if you don't have any past, how can you desire? What will you desire? To desire anything, experience, accumulated experience is needed. If you cannot desire you will be in a vacuum—tremendously beautiful emptiness.

Only the original mind is free from desires, so don't fight with desires. That fight will not lead you anywhere because to fight with desires you will have to create anti-desires. And they are as much desires as other desires. Don't fight with desires; see the fact. The original mind cannot be found through fighting with desires. You may find a better mind, but not the original mind. You may have a sinner's mind, and if you fight with it, you may gain a saint's mind; but the saint is nothing but sinner upside-down.

Sinners and saints are not separate beings; they are two aspects of the same coin. You can turn the coin this way or that. A sinner can become the saint any moment, and the saint can become the sinner any moment. And the sinner is always dreaming of becoming a saint, and the saint is always afraid of falling again back into the mire of sin. They are not separate; they exist together. In fact, if all sinners disappeared from the world, there will be no possibility for saints. They cannot exist without sinners.

I have heard: A priest was going to his church. On the way, by the side of the road, he saw a man who had been stabbed, almost dying. Blood was flowing. He rushed, but when he went near and saw the man's face, he shrank back. He knew this face well. This man was nobody else but the devil himself. He had a picture in his church of the devil. But the devil said, "Have compassion on me. And you talk about compassion, and you talk about love! And have you forgotten? Many times you have been preaching in your church, 'Love your enemy.' I am your enemy; love me."

Even the priest could not deny the validity of the argument. Yes, who is more an enemy than a devil? For the first time he became aware, but still he could not bring himself to help a dying devil. He said, "You are right, but I know that the devil can quote scriptures. You cannot befool me. It is good that you are dying. It is very good; the world will be better if you die." The devil laughed, a very devilish laugh and he said, "You don't know; if I die, you will be nowhere. You will have to die with me. And now I am not quoting scripture, I am talking business. Without me where will you be, and your church, and your God?" Suddenly, the priest understood. He took the devil on his shoulders and went to the hospital. He had to, because even God cannot exist without the devil.

Without the sinner, the saint cannot exist. They feed upon each other, they protect each other, they defend each other. They are not two separate things; they are two poles of the same phenomenon.

The original mind is not a mind. It is neither the mind of the sinner nor the mind of the saint. The original mind has no mind in it. It has no definition, no boundary. It is so pure that you cannot even call it pure, because to call anything pure you have to bring the concept of impurity in. Even that will contaminate it. It is so

pure, so absolutely pure that there is no point in saying that it is
pure.

*Only the original mind which is born of meditation
is free from desires.*

Now, *tatra dhyanajam*—'born out of meditation' is a literal
translation, but something is missed in it. Sanskrit is a very poetic
language. It is not just a language, it is not just a grammar; it is
more a poetry, a very condensed poetry. If it is rightly translated, if
the sense is translated and not only the letter, then I will translate
it 'which is re-born of meditation'; not just born, because the
original mind is not born. It is already there, just re-born; it
is already there, just re-cognized; it is already there, just re-
discovered. God is always a rediscovery. Your own being is already
there. It cannot be emphasized too much: it is already there; you
reclaim it. Nothing new is born, because the original mind is not
new, is not old; it is eternal, always and always and always.

Anasayam means: without any motivation, without any support,
without any cause, without any ground.

Tatra dhyanajam anasayam.

The original mind exists without any motivation. It exists without any cause. It exists without any support: *anasayam* literally
means without any support. It exists without any ground, ground-
less. It exists in itself, it has no outward support. It has to be so
because the ultimate cannot have any support—because the ultimate means the total—nothing is outside it. You can think that you
are sitting on the earth, and then the earth is being supported by
some magnetic forces in the planetary system, and the planets are
supported by some other magnetic force of some super-sun. But the
whole cannot have any support, because from where will the
support come? The total cannot have any grounding to it.

You go to the market; of course, you have a motivation: you go to
earn money. You come home; you have certain motivation: to rest.
You eat food because you are hungry; there is a cause to it. You
have come to me—there is a motivation; you are in search of
something. It may be vague, clear, known, not known, but the
motivation is there. But what can be the motivation of the total? It
is unmotivated, it is desireless—because motivation will bring
something from the outside. That's why Hindus call it *leela*, a play.
A play comes from the inside: you are just going for a walk—there

is no motivation, not even health. A health fanatic never goes for a walk; he cannot go because he cannot enjoy the very walk. He's calculating, "How many miles?" He's calculating, "How many deep breaths?" He's calculating, "How much perspiration?" He's calculating. He is taking the morning walk as work to be done, as an exercise. It is not just a play.

The English word 'illusion' is almost always used as a translation for the Eastern word 'maya'. Ordinarily, the word 'illusion' means unreal, but that is not its true meaning. It comes from a Latin root, *ludere*, which means to play. 'Illusion' simply means a play, and that is the real meaning of maya. Maya does not mean illusory; it simply means playful: God is playing with Himself. Of course, He was nobody except Himself, so He is playing a hide-and-seek with Himself. He hides one of His hands and tries to find it with another hand, knowing all the time where it is.

The original mind is unmotivated, with no cause. Other minds which are not original but imposed upon are, of course, motivated, and because of motivation we cultivate them. If you want to become a doctor you will have to cultivate a certain mind: you will have to become a doctor. If you want to become an engineer you will have to cultivate another sort of mind. If you want to become a poet, you cannot cultivate the mind of a mathematician. Then you will have to cultivate the mind of a poet. So whatsoever is your motivation, you create a certain mind.

I have heard: A lady was seated on a bus with her son. She bought a single ticket. The conductor addressed the boy, "How old are you, little fellow?"

"I am four," answered the lad.

"And when will you be five?" asked the conductor.

The boy glanced at his mother, who was smiling her approval of the conversation, and said, "When I get off this bus."

He has been taught to say something but still he cannot understand the motivation. He has been taught to say 'four years' to save a ticket, but he does not know the motivation of it so he repeats like a parrot.

Every child is more in tune with the original mind than grownups. Look at children, playing, running around: you will not find any motivation in particular. They are enjoying, and if you ask for what, they will shrug their shoulders. It is almost impossible to communicate with grown-ups. The children simply feel it almost impossible; there exists no bridge, because the grown-up asks a very silly question: "For what?" The grown-up lives with a certain economic mind. You do something to earn something. Children are not yet aware of this constant motivation. They don't know the language of desire, they know the language of playfulness. That's the meaning when Jesus says, "You will not be able to enter into the kingdom of God unless you are like small children." He's saying that unless you become a child again, unless you drop motivation and become playful. . . . Remember, work has never led anybody to God. And people who are working their path towards God will go on moving in a circle in the market-place; they will never reach Him. He is playful, and you have to be playful. Suddenly, communion; suddenly, a bridge.

Meditate playfully, don't meditate seriously. When you go into the meditation hall, leave your serious faces where you leave your shoes. Let meditation be fun. 'Fun' is a very religious word; 'seriousness' is very irreligious. If you want to attain to the original mind, you will have to live a very non-serious, though sincere life; you will have to transform your work into play; you will have to transform all your duties into love. 'Duty' is a dirty word; of course, a four-letter word.

Avoid duty. Bring more love to function. Change your work more and more into a new energy which you can enjoy, and let your life be more of a fun, more of a laughter, and less of desire and motivation. The more you are motivated, the more you will cling to a certain mind. You have to, because the motivation can be fulfilled only by a certain mind. And if you want to drop all mind—and all minds are to be dropped—only then do you attain to your innermost nature, your spontaneity. It is totally different, a different language from desire.

Let me tell you one anecdote.

There was a case against Mulla Nasrudin in the court. After hearing the early part of the evidence in a case brought before the County Court, the judge directed that the remainder of the case should be heard 'in camera'. Mulla Nasrudin, the defendant, objected on the grounds that he did not know the meaning of the word 'in camera', but the judge over-ruled the objections, saying, "I know what it means, the defending counsel knows what it means, the prosecution knows what it means, and the jury knows what it means; now clear the Court."

This having been done, counsel for the defense asked Mulla Nasrudin, the defendant, to tell the court in his own words what had happened on the night in question. "Well," said Mulla Nasrudin, "I was walking this girl home along a country lane and we

decided to take a short-cut across a field. Half-way across the field,
she seemed tired, so we sat down for a rest. It was a nice summer's
night and I felt a bit romantic, so I gave her a kiss, and she gave me
a kiss, and I gave her a kiss, and she gave me a kiss, and ten
minutes later, hi-tiddly-hi-tee."

The judge said, "Hi-tiddly-hi-tee?—what on earth does that
mean?"

"Well," answered Nasrudin, "the defending counsel knows what
it means, the prosecuting counsel knows what it means, and the
jury knows what it means—and if you had been there with your
camera, *you'd* know what it means!"

Desire has its own language, motivation has its own language,
and all languages are of desire and motivation—different desires.
Let me tell you this: Christianity is a language for a certain desire.
It is not religion. Hinduism is a language for some other desire, but
it is not a religion; and so on and so forth.

The original mind has no language. You cannot reach to it by
being a Hindu, a Christian, a Mohammedan, a Jaina, a Buddhist,
no. These are all desires. Through them you want to attain something. They are your greed projected.

The original mind is known when you drop all desiring, all
languages, all minds. And you suddenly don't know who you are. A
religious person is one who has dropped all his identity with any
pattern of thinking and is simply standing there naked, alone,
surrounded by existence without any dressing, without any cover-
ing of language and minds—an onion, peeled completely; emptiness has come into the hands.

Tatra dhyanajam anasayam.

Only the original mind which is born of meditation
is free from desires.

So how to attain to this original mind? Now, one of the most
important problems in religion has to be understood: the original
mind is free from desires, and the way to attain it is to become
desireless. A problem arises for the thinking intellect: what is
primary?—whether we have to drop the desires, and then can we
attain the original mind? But then the problem arises that if only
the desires are dropped when the original mind is attained, then
how can we drop desires before it is attained? Or, if the original
mind has to be attained, then desires drop of themselves, of their
own accord, as a consequence of it. Then we have to attain the

original mind when desires are still there, and the original mind cannot be attained without dropping desires, so a paradox arises. But the paradox is only because your intellect divides. In fact, the original mind and being desireless are not two things; it is just one phenomenon talked about in two ways. It is just one energy—call it desirelessness or call it the original mind—it is not two things. It happens simultaneously; I know.

Unless the original mind is attained you cannot become absolutely desireless, but you can become ninety-nine point nine per cent desireless, and that is the way. You start understanding your desires. Through understanding, many of them simply disappear because they are simply stupid. They have not led you anywhere except into more and more frustration. They have opened doors for hell and nothing else—more anguish, more anxiety, more pain and agony. Just look at them; they will disappear. First, desires which have led you into frustration will disappear, and then you will attain to a more keen perspective. Then you will see that desires which you have been thinking up to now, desires which have led you into pleasure, have also not led you into pleasure—because whatsoever seems to be pleasant finally, eventually, turns sour and bitter.

So pleasure seems to be a trick of desire: to trick you into pain. First the painful will drop, and then you will be able to see that the pleasure is illusory, unreal, a dream. Ninety-nine point nine per cent of desires will disappear through understanding, and then the final happens. It happens simultaneously: a hundred per cent of desires disappear, and the original mind arises in a single moment, not as cause and effect, but simultaneous, together.

It is better to use Carl Gustav Jung's term for it: synchronicity. They are not related as cause and effect. They appear together simultaneously, and that too has to be said that way because I have to use language. Otherwise they are one, two faces of the same coin. If you look through understanding, meditation, you will call it the original mind. If you look through your desires, passions, you will call it desirelessness. When you call it desirelessness it simply shows that you have been comparing it with desire; when you call it the original mind, it simply shows that you have been comparing it with the mechanical minds, but you are talking about one and the same thing.

Wherever you are, you are in a mechanical mind. Whoever you are, you are in a mechanical mind, imprisoned. Don't feel sorry for yourself. That's natural. Every child has to learn something; that creates mind. And every child has to learn ways to survive in the world; that creates the mind. Don't feel angry against your parents or against your society; that is not going to help. In love they have helped you; it was natural.

You needed a mind to survive, and every society tries to force every child because all children, as born, are wild. They have to be tamed, they have to be framed. They come frameless. It will be difficult for them to survive and live in a world where much struggle goes on, where survival is a continuous problem. They have to become efficient in certain ways to protect themselves. They have to be armoured, protected, sealed against the inimical forces in the world. They have to be taught to behave like others; they have to be taught to be imitative. The mechanical mind is created through imitation. The original mind is created by dropping imitation.

I have heard: Three ghosts were playing cards when a fourth ghost opened the door and came in. The draft from the outside blew all the cards on the floor. The new ghost was a child ghost—very young, very new to the world of the ghosts. One of the ghosts looked up and said, "Can't you use the keyhole like everybody else?"

Now even ghosts have to be trained: "There is no need to open the door; come through the keyhole as everybody is doing!"

That's how parents go on teaching you—imitate—and those who are great imitators are appreciated. A child who does not imitate is punished. A rebellious child is punished, an obedient child is praised. Obedience is thought to be a great value, and rebellion a great disvalue. The whole society tries to make you obedient, forces you: through awards, through punishments, fear, appreciation, ego-enhancement. There are a thousand and one ways to force you to just imitate others, because that is the only way to give you a frame, to give you a narrowness, to give you a tamed discipline. But of course, this is at a very great cost. It had to happen, it has happened, and there was no other way. Nobody could have avoided it, and I don't see that there will ever be a possibility of avoiding it completely. More or less, it will be there.

People ask me, if I had to teach children, what would I teach them? But whatsoever you teach them will give them a mind. You can teach them rebellion, but that too will give them a mind. They will start imitating the rebellious people. Again they will be framed.

Krishnamurti has a few schools around the world to teach children so that they don't become imitators—but they become imitators all the same. They start imitating Krishnamurti. The problem is very subtle. When you teach the children not to imitate, they start imitating you; they say, "Don't imitate!" You teach them that imitation is a disvalue, and of course, you use the same means. If they imitate they are condemned; everybody looks down upon them. If they become rebellious, they are appreciated. It is the same mechanism of award and punishment, of fear and greed. They become imitation rebels, but how can a rebel be an imitator?

There is no way to avoid the mind, but there is a way to come out of it. It has to be accepted as a necessary evil of being born in a society, of being born out of parents. It is a necessary evil to be tolerated. Of course, make it as loose as possible, that's all. Make it as liquid as possible, that's all. A good society is the society which gives you a mind, and yet keeps you alert that one day this mind has to be dropped—"This is not any ultimate value; it has to be gone through but gone beyond also. It has to be transcended." A mind has to be given, but there is no need to give an identity with the mind. If the identity remains a little relaxed, when people are grown up they will be able to come out of it more easily, with less pain, less agony, less effort.

Whether you are rich or poor, whether you are white or black, whether you are educated or uneducated, it makes no difference; we are in the same boat: the boat of the artificial mind. And that's the problem. So you can become rich from being poor, or you can renounce your riches and can become a beggar, a Buddhist *bhikkhu*, a monk, but that will not change you. You will still remain in the same boat. You will simply be changing roles. You will be changing personalities, but your essence will remain confined.

I have heard: The millionaire saw the old tramp wandering around his garden and shouted to him, "Get out of here this minute!" The tramp said, "Look here mister, the only difference between you and me is that you are making your second million, while I'm still working on my first"—not much of a difference.

The poor man, the rich man, the educated, the uneducated, the cultured, the uncultured, the civilized, the primitive, the Western, the Eastern, the Christian, the Hindu: it makes no difference. Differences may be of some quantity, but not of quality. We are all in the mind, and the whole of religion is an effort to get beyond it.

Karmasuklakrsnam yoginas tri-vidham itaresam.

The yogi's karmas are neither pure nor impure, but all others are three-fold: pure, impure, and mixed.

This is something which has been very, very difficult to be understood in the West, because in the West only two categories exist: pure and impure, the saintly and the sin, the divine and the devilish, heaven and hell, black and white. The whole West follows the Aristotelian logic, and it has not yet come to be aware of something transcendental which goes beyond both and is neither. Sutras like this are very difficult to be understood by a Western mind because the mind has a certain frame. The frame says, "How is it possible?—a man is either good or bad! How can a man be possible, a mind be possible which is neither?—you will be either good or bad." The dichotomy, the dualism is very clear in the Western mind. It is analytical.

The sutra says, "The yogi's karmas are neither pure nor impure because they come out of the original mind." Now, many things are implied here.

You see somebody dying and immediately, in the Aristotelian mind, a problem arises: if God is good, why death; if God is good, why poverty; if God is good, why cancer? If God is good, then everything has to be good. Otherwise, doubt arises. Then God cannot be. Or, if He is, then He cannot be good. And how can you call a God 'God' who is not even good? So the whole of Christian theology, for centuries, has been working out this problem; how to explain it away? But it is impossible—because with the Aristotelian mind it is impossible. You can avoid it, but you cannot completely dissolve it because it arises out of the very structure of that mind.

In the East we say that God is neither good nor bad, so whatsoever is happening, is happening. There is no moral value in it. You cannot call it good or bad. You call it such because you have a certain mind. It is in reference to your mind that something becomes good and something becomes bad.

Now look. . . . Adolf Hitler was born; if the mother had killed Adolf Hitler, would it have been good or bad? Now, we can see that if the mother had killed Adolf Hitler, it would have been very good for the world. Millions of people were killed; it would have been better to kill one person. But if the mother had killed Adolf Hitler she would have been punished tremendously. She might have been given a life sentence, or she might have been shot by the government, by the court, by the police. And nobody would have said that the government was wrong, because it is a sin to kill a child. But do you see the implications? Then Adolf Hitler killed millions of people. He had almost brought the world to the very verge of death. Nobody has been such a calamity ever before. All Genghis Khans' and Tamurlaines become pale before him. He was the greatest murderer ever. But what to say?—whether he did well or not is still difficult because life is never complete, and unless it is complete how can you evaluate it? Maybe whatsoever he did was good. Maybe he cleaned the earth of all wrong people—who knows? And who can decide it? Maybe without him the world would have been worse than it is.

Whatsoever we say is good is just according to a certain narrow mind. Whatsoever we say is bad is also according to a certain narrow mind.

There is a Taoist fable: A man had a very beautiful horse, so precious that even the emperor was envious and jealous. Many times offers had come to him, and people were ready to pay whatsoever amount of money he expected or asked. But the old man would laugh. He would say, "I love the horse and how can you sell your love? So thank you for your offer, but I cannot sell it."

Then one day, in the night the horse was stolen, or something happened. The horse was not found in the stable the next morning. The whole town gathered and they said, "Now look, silly old man!—the horse is gone. And you could have become very rich. Such a calamity has never happened in this town. And you are poor and old. You should have sold it; you did wrong."

The old man laughed. He said, "Don't go into evaluations, and don't say anything about good or bad, and don't talk about calamity or blessing. I know only one thing: that last night the horse was in the stable, this morning he is not there, that's all. But I don't say anything about it. Just remain with the fact: the horse is not in the stable—finished. Why bring any mind to it?—whether it is good or bad, whether it should not have happened, whether it is a calamity; forget all about it."

The people were shocked. They felt insulted that they had come to show their sympathy, and this fool was talking philosophy!—"So it has been good. This man needed to be punished, and Gods are always just."

But after fifteen days, the horse came back. It had not been stolen; it had escaped to the forest. And there came twelve other horses with it—wild horses, very beautiful, very strong. The whole town gathered. They said, "This old man knows something. . . . He was right; it was not a calamity. We were wrong." And they said, "We are sorry. We could not understand the whole situation, but it is a great blessing. Not only is your horse back, but twelve other horses! And we have never seen such beautifully strong horses. You will gather a lot of money."

The old man said again, "Don't bother about whether it is a blessing or a calamity. Who knows? Future is unknown, and we should not say anything unless we know the future. You are again making the same mistake. Just say, 'The horse is back, and is back with twelve other horses,' that's all." They said, "Now don't try to befool us. We know you have gathered a lot of money."

But after a week, the only son of the old man was teaching a horse, a wild horse, trying to tame it. He fell down from the horse. All over he was broken—many fractures. He was the only support of the old man, and the people said, "This old man knows, really knows . . . now this is a great calamity. This coming of the horse has been a misfortune. The only support in his old age, his son, is almost dead. He had been supporting the old man; now the old man will have to serve the young man because he will remain in the bed for his whole life. And he was just going to be married. Now the marriage will be impossible!"

And they gathered again, and again they spoke, and the old man said, "How to tell you? You go on doing the same thing again and again. Only say this much: that my young son has many fractures, that's all. Why move in the future? Why do you go so fast into the future? And you have seen for these few days that again and again you were wrong, but again and again you go off from the present and you start evaluating."

And it happened that after a few days, the country went to war with a neighboring country, and all the young men of the town were forcibly taken into the army. Only this old man's son was left because he had fractures. They again gathered, but before they gathered the old man said, "Keep quiet! When will you understand?—life is complex." This is the Eastern attitude, *in essence.*

The yogi lives in the original mind, in suchness. Whatsoever happens, happens; he never evaluates it. And he does not do anything on his own accord, he becomes just a vehicle of the whole. The whole flows through him. He becomes like a hollow bamboo, a flute. The yogi carries that which comes from God, from the total. That's why Krishna says to Arjuna in the Bhagavad-Gita, "Don't be worried, and don't think in terms that whatsoever you are going to do will be violence and you will kill so many people. If God wills so, let it be so. If He wants to kill, He will kill, whether through you or through somebody else. In fact," Krishna says, "He has already killed. You are just instrumental, so don't become too identified with your actions. Remain a witness."

The yogi's karmas are neither pure nor impure,
neither moral nor immoral, but all others are
three-fold: pure, impure, and mixed.

Whatsoever ordinary people are doing—by ordinary I mean people who have not attained to their innermost core of being; people who are living with their minds are ordinary, who are living with their ideas and thoughts and ideologies and scriptures, whatsoever they are doing—either their actions are pure, or their actions are impure, or their actions are mixed; but their actions are not spontaneous, not original. They react, they don't act. Their response is a reaction. It is not an overflowing of energy. They are not available to this moment, right now.

Somebody asked Lin Chi, a Zen Master, "If somebody comes and attacks you, what will you do?" He shrugged his shoulders. He said, "Let him come, and I will see. I cannot be prepared beforehand. I don't know. I may laugh, or I may weep, or I may jump and kill that man. Or, I may not bother about it at all. But I don't know. Let the man come. The moment will decide, not I. The whole will decide, not I. How can I say what I will do?"

An enlightened man does not live through the mind. He has no frame around him. He is vast emptiness. Nobody knows how God will act through him in that moment. He will not interfere—that's all—because there is nobody to interfere. Mind interferes; he is no more a mind. He will not try to do something which he thinks is good, and he will not try to avoid something which he thinks is bad. He will not try anything. He will be simply in the hands of the divine and let the thing happen. He will not interpret later on that whatsoever has happened is good or bad. No, an enlightened man never looks back, never evaluates, never looks ahead, never plans. Whatsoever the moment . . . and he allows the moment to decide. In that moment, everything converges. The whole existence takes part, so nobody knows.

Lin Chi said, "If somebody attacks me, nobody knows. It will depend. The somebody may be Gautam Buddha, and if he attacks me I will laugh. I may touch his feet at how compassionate it is of him to attack me, poor Lin Chi. But it will depend on the moment, on so many things that it is unpredictable."

Just at the beginning of this century, in the year 1900, a great scientist, Max Planck, came to make one of the greatest discoveries ever. He came to feel and he came to discover that existence seems to be discontinuous, that it is not a continuity. It is not as if you

pour oil from one pot into another. Then the oil has a continuity; it
falls in a continuous stream. Max Planck said, "Existence is such:
as if you are pouring peas from one carton into another—
discontinuous—each pea falling separately." He said, "The whole
life is discontinuous. These discontinuous elements he calls
'quanta'. That is his Theory of Quantum. 'Quanta' means: each
thing is separate from each other thing, and discontinuous, and
between two things there is a space. Now, that space is holding
everything because two things are not connected, two atoms are
not connected between themselves. The space, the emptiness is
holding both. They are not connected directly, they are connected
through space. Still, nobody has tried some parallel theory about
mind, but exactly the same is the case.

Two thoughts are not connected with each other, and thoughts
are discontinuous. One thought, another thought, another thought,
and between these thoughts, there are gaps, very small gaps—that
is your inner space. That's what original mind is. One cloud passes,
another cloud passes; between the two is the sky. One thought
passes, another passes; between the two is the original mind. If you
think your thoughts are continuous, then you think of yourself as a
mind.

In fact, there is nothing like a mind—only thoughts, discontinuous thoughts wandering within you, moving so fast that you cannot
see the gaps. These thoughts are held by your inner space. Atoms
are supported by the outer space, thoughts are supported by the
inner space. If you count matter, you become a materialist; if you
count your thoughts, you become a mentalist. But mind and matter, both are false. They are processes, discontinuous. And I would
like to say to you that this is yoga's ultimate synthesis: that the
inner space and the outer space are not two. Your original mind
and God's original mind are not two. Your artificial mind is different from God, but your original mind is nothing different. It is the
same.

> *Desires arise from these three-fold karmas when*
> *circumstances are favorable for their fulfillment.*

If you do a pure karma, a good act, a saintly act, then desires
will arise, of course, to do more good. If you do an impure act,
desires will arise to do more impure acts, because whatsoever you
do creates a certain habit in you to repeat it. People go on repeating. Whatsoever you have done, you become skillful in doing it. If

you do a mixed act, of course a mixed desire arises in which good and bad are both mixing. But all are artificial minds. Even the mind of the saint is still a mind.

I have heard:

Abe Cohen, a great businessman, a Jew, was convicted of murder before the ending of capital punishment. The prison governor visited him on the morning of his execution. "Mr. Cohen," he said, "it will cost this country 100 pounds to hang you." "Bad business," said Abe. "Give me 95 pounds, and I will shoot myself."

A businessman is a businessman. He goes on thinking in terms of business, in terms of money. He has become skillful about it. Just watch whatsoever you have been doing—you have a tendency to repeat it, unawares, unconsciously. You go on repeating the same things again and again and again, and of course, the more you repeat, the more you are caught in the habit. A time comes when even if you want to leave the habit, the habit has become so deep-rooted that you want to leave it, but it does not want to leave you.

I have heard, it happened: A certain teacher, out of indigence, wore only thin cotton cloth in the winter. A storm carried a bear down from the mountains by way of the river. Its head was hidden in the water. The children, seeing its back, cried, "Teacher, look! A fur coat has fallen into the water, and you are cold. Go and fetch it!" The teacher, in the extremity of his need, leapt into the river to catch the fur coat. The bear quickly attacked him and caught him. "Teacher," the boys shouted from the bank, "either grasp the coat, or let it go and come out!" "I am letting the fur coat go," shouted the teacher, "but the fur coat is not letting me go!"

That's the problem with habits: first you cultivate them, then, by and by, they have become almost a second nature to you. Then you want to drop them, but it is not so easy to drop them. What to do?

You will have to become more aware.

Habits cannot be dropped. There are only two ways to drop them: one is to change the habit for a substitute habit—but that is just changing one problem for another, it is not going to help much; the other is to become more aware. Whenever you repeat a habit, become aware. Even if you have to repeat it, repeat it, but repeat with a witnessing, an alertness, an awareness. That awareness will make you separate from the habit, and the energy that you go on giving to the habit unknowingly, will not be given anymore. By and by, the habit will shrink; the water will not be flowing through it, the channel will be blocked. By and by, it will disappear.

Never try to change one habit into another, because all habits are bad. Even good habits are bad, because they are habits. Don't try to change impure habits into pure habits. It is good for the society that you change your bad habits into good habits. Rather than going to the pub every day, if you go to the church or to the temple every day, it is good for the society. But as far as you are concerned it is not going to help much. You have to go beyond habits. Then it is helpful.

The society wants you to become moral, because by being immoral you create troubles—society is finished. Once you become moral, the society is finished. Now it is none of the society's business to be bothered with you. If you are immoral, the society is not finished with you; something has to be done about you. Once you are moral, the society is finished. The society garlands you and cheers you and says, "You are a very good man"—finished. The society is no more in trouble with you, but you yourself have yet long to go; the journey is not complete yet. The bad habit is against society, and habit, as such, is against your original nature.

A flea rushed into the pub just before closing time, ordered five double scotches, drank them straight down, rushed into the street, leapt high in the air and fell flat on his face. He picked himself up, looked unsteadily around and muttered, "Darn it! Someone has moved my dog."

For many lives you have been drinking and drinking out of unconsciousness. Everybody is an alcoholic, and of course you go on falling again and again.

The deep problem is: how to become aware, how not to be unconscious. From where to start? Don't try to fight with some very deep-rooted habit. You will be defeated. The fur coat will not leave you so easily. Start with very neutral habits.

For example: you go for a walk; just be aware that you are walking. It is a neutral thing. Nothing is invested in it. You are looking at the trees; just look at the trees and be aware. Don't look with clouded eyes. Drop all thinking. Just for a few moments even, just look at the trees, and *just* look. Look at the stars. Swimming, just be alert to the inner feeling that happens inside your body while you are swimming, the inner. Feel it. You are taking a sun bath; feel how you start feeling inside: warm, settled, rested. While falling asleep, just watch how you are feeling inside. Inside, outside—try to be aware of the coolness of the sheets, the darkness in the room, the silence outside, or the noise outside. Suddenly, a dog barks—neutral things; bring your consciousness to them first. And then, by and by, proceed.

Then, try to be aware of your good habits, because good habits
are not so deep-rooted as bad habits. Good habits need much
sacrifice on your part, so very few people try to cultivate good
habits. And even those who try to cultivate good habits try very few
good habits; just underneath, many bad habits are there.

First try neutral, then good, then move by and by to bad habits.
And finally, remember that each habit has to be made aware. Once
you have become aware of your whole habitual pattern, that
habitual pattern is your mind. Any day the shift will happen.
Suddenly, you will be in the no-mind. When all the habits of your
life have become aware, you don't do them unconsciously and you
don't cooperate with them unconsciously, any day, when the satu-
ration point comes—at one hundred degrees—suddenly, a shift
will happen. You will find yourself in emptiness. That is the original mind which is neither pure nor impure.

> *Desires arise from these three-fold karmas when*
> *circumstances are favorable for their fulfillment.*

Whatsoever you do remains like a seed in you. And whenever a
certain circumstance arises which can be helpful to you, the seed
sprouts. Sometimes we carry seeds for many lives. The right circumstance, the right season may not be come across, but whenever
it comes it creates very complex problems. Suddenly, you come
across a man on the road and you feel very, very repelled, and you
have not ever known the man. You have not even thought about
him, heard about him; an absolute stranger, and suddenly you feel
repelled, or, you feel attracted. Suddenly you feel as if you have met
him before. Suddenly you feel as if a deep surge of love-energy is
arising in you for this stranger, as if you have been always close,
always close. A seed has been carried from some other life—a
certain circumstance—and that seed starts sprouting. Suddenly,
you are miserable for no reason at all. And you think, "Why am I
miserable? Why?" There seems to be no cause in the visible world.
You may be carrying a seed for this misery; just a right moment
has arrived.

Julia came to her father with her head downcast. "Poppa," she
said, "you know that rich Mr. Wolfe? Well, he betrayed me, and I
am going to have a baby."

"My God!" said the father. "Where is he? I will kill him! Give me
his address. I will murder him!" Dashing to the rich man's home,
he cornered him and in a loud voice told him what he intended to

do. But the rich Mr. Wolfe was quite calm. "Don't get excited," he
said. "I am not running away, and I intend to do right by your
daughter. If she has a boy, she gets $50,000; if it is a girl, she gets
$35,000. Is that fair?"

The father halted, while the look of anger on his face changed.
"And if it is a miscarriage," he pleaded, "will you give her another
chance?"

Suddenly, the circumstances had changed. Now a seed of greed
sprouts. He had come to murder, but just the mention of money
and he had forgotten all about murder; he's asking, "Will you give
her another chance?"

Watch . . . watch yourself continuously; circumstances change
and you immediately change. Something in you starts sprouting,
something starts closing.

The man of original mind remains the same. Whatsoever happens, he watches it, but there are no longer any seeds of desire left
from the past. He does not act through his past, he simply responds; out of nothingness comes his response. Sometimes you also
act in that way, but very rarely. And whenever you act that way,
you feel a tremendous fulfillment and satisfaction and contentment.
It happens sometimes.

Somebody is dying, drowning in the river, and you simply jump
without any thought. You don't think whether to save this man or
not, whether he is a Hindu or a Mohammedan, or a sinner or a
saint, or why you should be worried. No, you don't think. Suddenly,
it happens. Suddenly, your mind is pushed away and your original
mind acts. And when you get that man out, you feel tremendous
contentment, as you have never felt before. A harmony arises in
you. You feel very fulfilled. Whenever something out of your nothingness happens, you feel blissful.

Bliss is a function of your nothingness.

*Because memories and impressions retain the same
form, the relationship of cause and effect continues
even though separated by class, locality, and time.*

And it goes on . . . your life changes: you die in this body, you
enter into another womb, but the innermost form clings with you.
Whatsoever you have done, desired, experienced, accumulated, that
fur coat clings with you; you carry it with you. The death, ordinary
death, is only the death of the body; the mind continues. The real
death, the ultimate death we call samadhi, is not only the death of

the body; it is the death of the mind as such. Then there is no more birth, because then there is no seed left to come back to, no desire left to be fulfilled. Nothing left, one simply disappears like a fragrance. . . .

And there is no beginning to this process as the desire to live is eternal.

Philosophers go on asking, "When did this world start?" Yoga says a very tremendous thing: the world has never started. The desire has no beginning, because to desire to live is eternal. It has been always there. Yoga does not believe in any creation. It is not that God created the world on some day, at some moment. No, desire has been always there. There was no beginning for desire, but there is an end to it. This has to be understood. It is very illogical, but if you understand you will be able to feel the point.

Desire has no beginning, but it has an end. Desirelessness has a beginning, but has no end; and the circle is complete. Desire has no beginning but has an end. If you become aware, the end comes, and *then* starts desirelessness. Desirelessness has a beginning, but then there is no end to it. "The world has no beginning"; we have been saying in the East, "it has continued always and always; but it has an end." For a Buddha, it ends. Then it is no longer there. Just like a dream, it disappears. But the no-world—*nirvana, kaivalya, moksha*—that has a beginning but no end. So we never ask when the world started. We have not bothered about it because it has never started.

We have not paid much attention to the birth dates of Krishna, Buddha, Mahavir, but we have paid much attention to the day that they attained enlightenment—because that is the real beginning of something which is never going to end. The enlightenment day of Buddha is very significant; that we have remembered, that we have worshipped again and again, again and again. Nobody knows when he was born; nobody has bothered about it. In fact, the myth says that he was born on the same day as the day he died, and he became enlightened also on the same day. My feeling is, we have forgotten his birthday and his death day; we remember only his enlightenment day. But only that is significant: that his birthday was also his death day, because that is the only significant thing that happens in a life—the beginning of the endless.

Desire has no beginning, has been always here, but it can end. Desirelessness can begin and will never end. And between desire and desirelessness, the circle is complete. It is the same energy. That which has been desire becomes desirelessness. It is the same energy. And of course, desirelessness never ends. A man who has attained has become liberated, never comes back, because evolution cannot go backwards. There is no way to go backwards. Higher and higher we go, until the ultimate is attained. But from that, there is no point of falling back.

And there is no beginning to this process as the
desire to live is eternal.

Try to be aware of your desire because that has been your life up to now. Don't be caught in it. Try to understand it. Don't try to fight also, because that is again getting caught in it in another way. Just try to understand it: how it grips you, how it enters into you and makes you absolutely unconscious.

I have heard: "Abe, I have a wonderful bargain for you. I can get an elephant for $200." "But Izzy, don't be an idiot. What am I going to do with an elephant?"

"What are you going to do with an elephant? Don't be an idiot yourself! Think of the bargain. Where can you pick up an elephant for $200, tell me?"

"But I have a two-room flat. Where am I going to put an elephant?"

"What is the matter with you? Don't you recognize a bargain when you see one? As a matter of fact, I have even better news for you. If you want, I can get you two elephants for $300."

"Ah, now you are talking."

Now a man who has only a two-room flat has forgotten completely.

Watch desire. It goes on befooling you; it goes on leading you astray. It goes on leading you into illusions, into dreams.

Watch.

Before you take a step, watch, be alert. And by and by, you will see desires disappear, and the energy that was invested in desires is released. Millions are the desires, and when the energy is released from all those desires you become a tremendous upsurge of energy. You start soaring high. Naturally, the energy goes on pooling inside. The level of energy goes higher and higher, and one day, you start overflowing from *sahasrar*. You become a lotus, a one-thousand-petalled lotus.

CHAPTER FOUR
May 4, 1976

EVERYTHING IS
INTERDEPENDENT

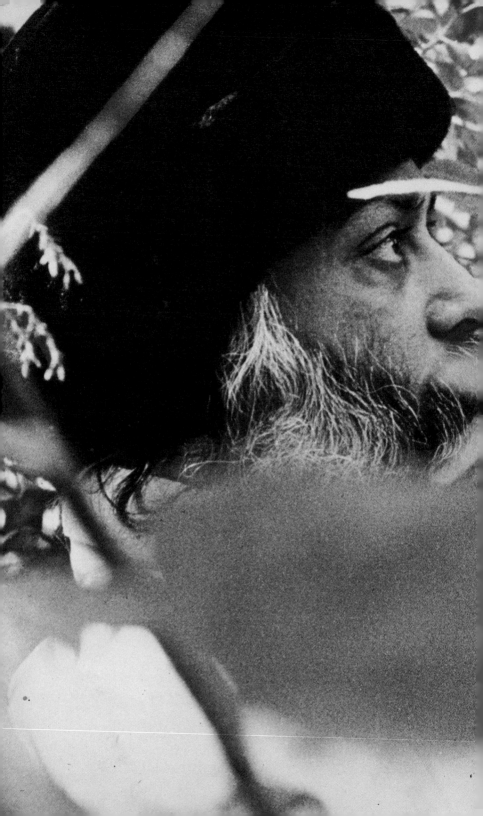

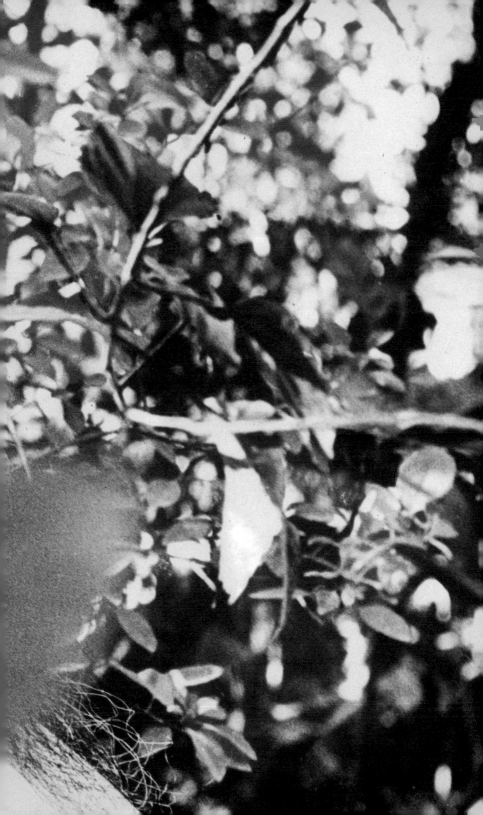

The first question:

While talking about wisdom, insights, and enlightenment, you often say 'we in the East'. Please explain the meaning of this phrase.

THE EAST HAS NOTHING TO DO WITH THE EAST. The East is just symbolic of the inner space, of the inner world of consciousness. East is symbolic of religion, West is symbolic of science. So even if in the East a person attains to a scientific attitude, he becomes Western. He may live in the East, he may be born in the East—that doesn't matter. Or, whenever a person attains to religious consciousness—he may be born in the West, it makes no difference—he begins to be a part of the East. Jesus, Francis, Eckhart, Boehme, Wittgenstein, even Henry Thoreau, Emerson, Swedenborg—they are all Eastern. The East is symbolic, always remember. I am not concerned with geography. So whenever I say 'we in the East', I mean all who have come to know the inner reality. And whenever I say 'you in the West', I simply mean the scientific mind, the technological mind, the Aristotelian mind: rational, mathematical, scientific, but not intuitive; objective but not subjective.

Once you understand it, then there will be no problem. All the great religions were born in the East. The West has not yet produced a great religion. Christianity, Judaism, Mohammedanism, Hinduism, Jainism, Buddhism, Tao: they were all produced in the East. It is something like a feminine mind, and it has to be so because on every level there is a meeting of *yin* and *yang*, the male and the female. The circle has to be divided. The East functions as a feminine part, the West functions as a male part.

The male mind is aggressive; science is aggressive. The feminine mind is receptive; religion is receptive. Science tries hard. It forces nature to reveal its secrets. Religion simply waits, prays and waits, invokes but does not force; calls, cries, weeps, persuades, almost seduces nature to reveal its mysteries and secrets, but the effort is feminine. Hence, meditation. When the effort is male, aggressive, it is like the laboratory: all sorts of instruments to torture nature, to force nature to reveal its secrets, to hand over the key. The male mind is an attack. The male mind is a rapist mind, and science is a rape. Religion is the mind of a lover; it can wait. It can wait infinitely.

So whenever I say 'we in the East', I mean all, wherever they were born, wherever they were brought up. They are spread all over the world. The East is spread all over the world, just as the West is spread all over the world. When somebody from India gets a Nobel prize for his scientific discoveries, he is a Western mind. He's no more part of the East, he's no more part of the Eastern tradition. He has changed his home, he has changed his address. Now he has fallen in line, in the queue with Aristotle.

The East is within you, and we call it 'East' because East is nothing but the rising sun: awareness, consciousness, alertness.

So never be confused whenever I say 'we in the East'. I don't mean the countries that are in the East, no. I mean the consciousness that is Eastern. I don't mean India when I use the word 'India'. It is a bigger thing for me. It is not just on the map as other countries. It is simply symbolic of the tremendous energy that India has put into the inner search. So wherever you are born, if you start moving towards God, you become Indian. Suddenly, your pilgrimage towards India starts. You may come to India or you may not come; that is not the point. But you have started your pilgrimage. And the day you realize, suddenly you will become part of Gautam Buddha, Mahavir the Jaina, the Upanishadic seers, the rishis of the Vedas, Krishna, Patanjali. Suddenly, you are no more part of the technological mind, the logical mind; you have become supra-logical.

The second question:

Jesus Christ, Buddha, Mahavir, Lao Tzu: all those enlightened have been known to go around the world preaching. Why is it that you are not doing the same?

I am doing the same, but just the other way round. I am allowing the world to come around me. This is my way. Buddha has done his thing, I am doing my thing.

The third question:

It is from Prem Madhuri.

I am often one of the crocodiles of which you speak, and sure enough, Bodhi shows every sign of becoming one of the great philosophers. That's fine, but what of the consciousness of the wretched crocodile?

The woman has suffered long because the feminine mind has suffered long. The woman has been oppressed long because the feminine mind has been oppressed long. Centuries upon centuries of oppression, exploitation, suppression; much violence has been done against women. Naturally, she has become cunning. Naturally, she has become very clever in devising subtle methods to torture men. That is natural. That is the way of the weak. Nagging, bitching—that is the way of the weak. Unless you understand it, you will not be able to drop it.

Why do women go on continuously nagging men, continuously finding ways and means to torture them? It is unconscious. It is centuries of repression that have poisoned their being, and of course, they cannot attack directly. That is not possible for many reasons. One: they are more fragile than man. They may learn karate, aikido, judo, but that will not make much difference. They are fragile; that is their beauty. If they learn too much karate and judo and ju-jitsu and aikido and become very muscular and strong, they will lose something—they will not gain. They will lose their femininity, they will lose their flower-like fragility, delicacy. That is not worth the effort.

Woman is fragile. She's meant to be that way. She has a deeper harmony than man. She's more musical, more rhythmic than man, more rounded. One thing: because of her fragileness she could not be as aggressive as man. Another thing: man has been training her in a certain way; man has been giving her a certain mind which does not allow her to move out of her bondage. It has been so long that it has reached to her very bones. She has accepted it. But freedom is such a thing that whatsoever happens, you remain freedom-oriented. You can never lose the desire to be free, because that is the desire to be religious, that is the desire to be divine. Freedom remains the goal, whatsoever happens.

So, what to do when there is no way to revolt and the whole society is that of man? How to fight it? How to protect a little dignity? So woman has become cunning and diplomatic. She starts doing things which are not directly an attack, but indirect. She fights with man in subtle ways. That has made her almost a crocodile. She waits continuously for her opportunity to take revenge. She may not be aware of anything in particular that she is fighting against, but she is just a woman, and she represents all womanhood. Centuries and centuries of indignities and humiliation are there. Your man may not have done anything wrong to you, but he is the representative of all men. You cannot forget it. You love the man, this man, but you cannot love the organization that men have created. You can love this man, but you cannot forgive man as such. And whenever you look into this man, you find the male mind there, and you start.

This is very unconscious. This creates a certain neurosis in women. More women are neurotic than men. It is natural, because they live in a man-made society, tailored for men, and they have to fit into it. It is tailored by men for men, and they have to live in it, they have to fit into it. They have to cut many of their parts, their limbs—alive limbs—to fit into the mechanical role that is given to them by man. They resist, they fight, and a certain neurosis arises out of this continuous fight. This is what bitching is.

I have heard: A sweet old lady went to a pet shop. Just in the shop window was a very beautiful dog, and she said to the shop owner, "That nice, sweet dog you have in the shop window?"

He said, "Yes lady, a very beautiful bitch. Isn't she beautiful?"

The woman was enraged. She said, "What! Watch your tongue! Don't use such words. This is a respectable part of the town. Be a little more cultured!"

Even the shop owner was a little puzzled, embarrassed. He said, "Sorry, but have you never heard the word used before?"

The lady said, "I have heard it used before, but never for a sweetie, sweet doggie!"

It is always used for women.

Just the other day I was reading a book called *Bitching*, written of course by a woman.

Something has gone very, very wrong. It is not a question of one woman, it is a question of womanhood. But by bitching and nagging and constant quarrelling, it cannot be remedied. That is not a remedy for it. Understanding is needed.

The question is certainly right. Madhuri is a crocodile, and she is doing much nagging and quarrelling with Bodhi. Of course, Bodhi is growing out of it. He has changed a lot. The whole credit goes to

Madhuri. When you have to live with a woman continuously
fighting and nagging, either you escape or you become a
philosopher, that is certain. Only two ways are available: either
you escape, or you start thinking that this is just *maya*, dream,
illusion: "This Madhuri is nothing but a dream. . . ." You become
detached. That is also a way of escaping. You remain there physi-
cally, but spiritually you go far away. You create a distance. You
hear the sounds Madhuri is making, but as if on some other planet.
Let her do; by and by, you become detached; by and by, you
become indifferent. For Bodhi it has been good.

Now, Madhuri is asking, "That's fine for Bodhi, but what of the
consciousness of the wretched crocodile?" Do the same as Bodhi is
doing. What is he doing? He's becoming more and more of a
watcher. He is not offended at what you are saying and doing. Even
if you are hitting him, he will watch it, as if something natural is
happening: old leaves are falling from the trees—what to do? A dog
is barking—what to do? It is night and it is dark—what to do? One
accepts, and in that acceptance one watches whatsoever is happening. Do the same. Just as Bodhi is watching you, you also watch
yourself. Because that crocodile is not your inner essence. No, it is
nobody's inner essence. That crocodile is just out of the wounds
that you are carrying in your mind, and those wounds have nothing
to do with Bodhi. Those wounds may have been done by somebody
else or may not have been done by anybody in particular, but just
by society.

Watch when you start behaving in a neurotic way, in a neurotic
style. Watch it!

Just as Bodhi is watching you, you also watch yourself.

And a distance will arise, and you will be able to see your own
mind creating unnecessary trouble. You will gather an awareness.
Continuously watching things, one gets out of the mind, because
the watcher is beyond the mind.

If you don't do that, the possibility is that as Bodhi grows more
and more philosophical and understanding, you will become more
and more of a bitch—because you will think that he is becoming
cold, you will think he is getting far away, and you will start hitting
him harder, you will start fighting harder. Seeing that he is going
somewhere else, leaving you, you will take more and more revenge.
Before it happens, become alert.

I have heard: A man arranged to pay for his wife's funeral
arrangements by installments, but after a few months he ran into
financial difficulties and was unable to keep up the payments.

Finally, the undertaker rang up one morning and said, "Look, either I get some money from you at once, or up she comes!"

Don't create such a situation that one who loves you starts thinking of your death, one who would have liked you to be immortal starts hoping that you die, that it is better that you die.

Mulla Nasrudin is mad after movies. Every night he's in the moviehouse, somewhere or other. One day the wife said, "I think that even if for one night you are at home, I will drop dead." He looked at her and he said, "Don't try to bribe me."

Don't create such a situation.

The wife of one of the club's oldest and more revered members had recently passed away. His fellow members were offering their condolences, and one said, "It is hard to lose one's wife...." Another member muttered bitterly, "Hard? It is damned near impossible!"

Nobody says this, but this is what people create—a very ugly situation. And I know that you are creating it unknowingly, and I know that you are creating it in the hope of just the opposite. Sometimes it happens that the woman starts hitting the man just to break his coolness, just to break the ice. She wants him to at least be warm: "At least be angry, but be warm. Hit me back, but do something! Don't stand there so aloof." But the more you create such a situation, the more the man has to protect himself and go far away. By and by, he has to learn space travel, so that the body remains here and he goes off far away—astral travel.

These are vicious circles. You want him to be close and warm and hugging you, but you create such a situation in which it becomes more and more impossible. Just watch what you are doing. And this man has not done anything in particular to you. He has not harmed you. I know there are situations where two persons don't agree, but that is part of growth. You cannot find a person who is going to agree totally with you. Particularly men and women don't agree because they have different minds, they have totally different attitudes about things. They function from different centers. So it is absolutely natural that they don't agree easily, but nothing is wrong with it. And when you accept a person and you love a person, you also love his or her disagreements. You don't start fighting, you don't start manipulating; you try to understand the other's point of view. And even if you cannot agree, you can agree to disagree. But still, a deep, subtle agreement remains that, "Okay, we agree to disagree. On this point we will not be coming to an agreement—right—but there is no need to fight." The fight is not going to bring you closer; it will create more distance. And much, almost ninety-five per cent of your quarrelling, is absolutely baseless; it is mostly misunderstanding. And we are so much fogged in our own heads that we don't give an opportunity to the other to show his mind.

In this too women have become very, very afraid. The problem, again, is of the male and female mind. Man is more argumentative. This much women have learned: that if you go through argumentation, he will win. So they don't argue, they fight. They get angry, and what they cannot do through logic, they do through anger. They substitute with anger, and of course, the man, thinking, "Why create so much trouble for such a small thing?" agrees. But this is not an agreement, and it will function as a block between the two.

Listen to his argument. There are possibilities that he may be right—because half of the world, the outer world, the objective world, has to be approached through reason. So whenever it is a question of the outer world, there is more possibility that the man may be right. But whenever it is a question of the inner world, it is more possible that the woman may be right because there, reason is not needed. So if you are going to purchase a car listen to the man, and if you are going to choose a church, listen to the woman. But it is almost impossible. If you have a wife you cannot choose your car—almost impossible. She will choose it. Not only that, she will sit at the back and drive it.

Man and woman have to come to a certain understanding that as far as the world of objects and things is concerned, man is more prone to be right and accurate. He functions through logic; he is more scientific, he is more Western. When a woman functions intuitively she is more Eastern, more religious. It is more possible that her intuition will lead her to the right path. So if you are going to a church, follow your woman. She has a more accurate feeling for things which are of the inner world. And if you love a person, by and by, you come to this understanding, and a tacit agreement arises between two lovers: who's going to be right in what.

And love is always understanding.

Two monsters from outer space were walking along the street when they saw a traffic signal. "I think she likes you," said the first monster. "One is winking at you." Just then the signal changed from go to stop. "Just like a woman," muttered the second monster, "can't make up her mind from one moment to the next."

It is very difficult for a woman to make up her mind because she is more fluid, more of a process, less of a solidity. That is her beauty and grace. She is more river-like, goes on changing. Man is more solid, more square, more certain, decisive. So where decisions are needed, listen to Bodhi, Madhuri. And when decisions are not needed, but floating, drifting is needed, then you can help Bodhi to listen to you; and he will listen.

The feminine mind can reveal many mysteries, as the male mind can reveal many mysteries; but as there is a conflict between science and religion, so is the conflict between man and woman. One day it is hoped that man and woman will come to complement each other rather than conflict with each other, but that day will be the same day as when science and religion also complement each other. Science will listen with understanding to what religion is saying, and religion will listen with understanding to what science is saying. And there is no trespass, because the fields are absolutely different. Science moves outward, religion moves inward.

Women are more meditative, men are more contemplative. They can think better. Good; when thinking is needed, listen to the man. Women can feel better. When feeling is needed, listen to the women. And both feeling and thinking make a life whole. So if you are really in love, you will become a yin/yang symbol. Have you seen the Chinese yin/yang symbol? Two fish are almost meeting and merging into each other in a deep movement, completing the circle of energy. Man and woman, female and male, day and night, work and rest, thinking and feeling: these are not antagonistic to each other, they are complementary. And if you love a woman or a man, you both are enhanced tremendously in your beings. You become complete.

That's why I say that Hindu concepts of God are more complete than Christian, Jewish, Mohammedan, or Jaina concepts; but both are concepts. Mahavir stands alone; no woman is to be found anywhere around. It is just a male mind, alone; the complementary is missing. Only one fish is in the circle, the other fish is not there. It is a half circle, and a half circle is not a circle at all because to call a circle 'half' is almost absurd. A circle has to be full; only then is it a circle. Otherwise, it is not a circle at all.

The Christian God is alone; no concept of female around Him. Something is missing. That's why the Christian or Jewish God is much too male, revengeful, angry, ready to destroy for small sins, ready to throw people into hell forever—no compassion, very hard, rock-like. The Hindu concept of God is closer to reality; it is a circle. Ram you will see with Sita; Shiva you will see with Devi; Vishnu you will see with Laxmi—always the complementary is there. Hindu Gods are more human compared to other Gods, which are almost inhuman. Hindu Gods are almost as if belonging to you, just amidst you, just like you—more pure, more whole, but connected to you. They are not disconnected; they are connected to your life experience.

Let love be your prayer also. Watch! Watch the crocodile in you and drop it, because that crocodile will not allow you to flower in deep love. That will destroy you, and destruction never fulfils anybody. Destruction frustrates. Fulfillment is only out of deep creativity.

A meek little man was just returning home from his wife's funeral. As he arrived at his front door, a chimney pot fell off the roof of the house and gave him a sharp blow on the back. Glancing up he muttered, "Ah . . . she has arrived already." Don't create such images of you in the mind of one who loves you.

And man needs much from a woman to grow: her love, her compassion, her warmth. The Eastern understanding about man and woman is this: that a woman is essentially a mother. Even a small girl is essentially a mother, a growing mother. Motherhood is not something that happens as an accident, it is a growth in a woman. Fatherhood is just a social formality; it is not necessary. It is not natural, in fact. It exists only in a human society; man has created it. It is an institution. Motherhood is not an institution, fatherhood is. A man has no inner necessity to be a father.

When a man falls in love with a woman, he is seeking a beloved. When a woman falls in love with a man, she is seeking someone who will make her a mother. She is seeking someone who she would like to become the father of her children. That's why when a woman tries to find a man her criterion is different; strong, because she will need protection and the children will need protection; rich, because she will need protection and the children will need protection. When a man is finding a woman, he is only concerned with a wife. His concern is with a beautiful woman whom he can enjoy and be with. He's not too concerned about being a father. If he becomes a father, that is accidental. If he starts liking it also, that also is accidental, because he likes the woman and the children have come out of her. He loves the children through the woman, and the woman loves the man through the children. Of course, it has to be so; the circle becomes complete. A woman is essentially a mother, in search of being a mother.

So the Eastern concept is that the woman is in search of being a mother, and the man is in search, deep down, of finding his lost mother. He has lost the womb of the mother, the warmth of the mother, the love of the mother. He is searching again for the woman who can become his mother.

Man essentially is a child. Even the very grown-up seventy or ninety-year-old man is a child. And a very small girl essentially is a mother. This is how the circle completes.

In the East, in the days of the Upanishads, the seers used to bless new couples with a very absurd idea. It will look absurd to the Western eye. They used to say, "God should give you ten children, and finally, the ultimate fulfillment of becoming a mother to your husband also." So in all, eleven children: ten children from the husband, and finally, the husband also becomes a child to you— eleven children. A woman is fulfilled when the husband also becomes a child to her.

Man goes on seeking his mother. When a man falls in love with a woman, he falls in love again with his mother. Somehow, this woman gives an idea of his mother. The way she walks, the face she has, the color of her eyes or the color of her hair, or her sound; something that gives the idea of the mother again. The warmth of her body, the care that she shows about him is a search for the lost mother. It is a search for the womb.

Psychoanalysts say that the male urge to penetrate the woman's body is nothing but the urge to again reach to the womb. It is meaningful. The very effort of man to penetrate the woman's body is nothing but an effort to reach the womb. Once you understand what is happening between your energy and your man's energy, what is really going on, watch it. By and by, the energy will start falling in a circle.

And help each other. We are together to help each other, to make each other happy and blissful, and finally, to give an opportunity through the meeting of man and woman for God to happen. Love is fulfilled only when it becomes samadhi. If it is not samadhi yet and the nagging and conflict and bitching continues, and fighting and anger, and this and that, then your love will never become a harmonious whole. You will never find God, which can be found only in love.

The fourth question:

Interdependence is a nice concept, but how is that possible when you urge all of us to be totally selfish?

First, interdependence is not 'nice', and it is not a concept.

It is not nice at all. Independence feels nice; dependence feels very, very bitter; interdependence is neither nice nor bitter. It is a very balancing thing: neither this way nor that. It leans to no side; it is a tranquility. And it is not a concept, it is a reality. It is how it is. Just watch life and you will never find anything which is not interdependent. Everything that exists, exists in the ocean of interdependence. It is not a concept, it is not a theory. You just drop all theories, all prejudices, and look at life.

Look at a small tree, a rose bush, and you will see the whole existence converges on it. From the earth it is connected. Without the earth, it would not be there. It goes on breathing the air. It is connected with the atmosphere. From the sun it goes on getting energy. The rose is rosy because of the sun, and these are very visible things. Those who have been working hard say that there are invisible influences also. They say that it is not only that the sun is giving energy to the rose, because nothing can be one way in life. The traffic cannot be one way. Otherwise, it would be a very unjust life. The rose would go on getting and giving nothing. No, it must be that the rose is also giving something to the sun. Without the rose, the sun would also miss something. That has yet to be discovered by science, but occultists have always felt that life is a give and take. It cannot be one way. Otherwise, the whole balance would be lost. The rose must be giving something—maybe a certain joy. Certainly, it gives fragrance to the air, and certainly it must be giving some creativity, a situation for the earth to be creative. The earth must be feeling happy through it; it has created a rose. It must be feeling fulfilled. A deep satisfaction and contentment must be coming to the earth.

Everything is connected. Nothing is unconnected here. So when I say interdependence, I don't mean that it is a concept, a theory, no.

Independence is a concept because it is absolutely false. Nobody has ever seen anything independent. An absolute dependence is false because nobody has ever seen anything absolutely dependent.

A child is born: you think he is completely helpless and dependent on the mother? Can't you see that the mother is also gaining much from him? In fact, the day the child is born, the mother is also born as a mother. Before it, she was just a plain woman. Now, something tremendously new has happened to her with the birth of the child. She has attained to motherhood. It is not only that the child is dependent on the mother, the mother is also dependent. You will see a certain grace happening to the woman when she becomes a mother, a certain harmony happening to her. If the mother dies, of course, the child will not be able to survive. But if the child dies, do you think that the mother will be able to survive? No, the mother will die. Again there will be a woman; the mother-hood will disappear with the child. And this woman will be less than she was before the child had happened to her. She will always miss something; a part of her being has disappeared with the child. That missing part will function as a wound continuously.

Everything is interdependent.

The tree goes on eating the earth, it goes on giving you fruit; you go on eating the fruit. Then you die, and the earth eats you, and the tree again eats the earth. And the fruit?—your grandchildren will be eating you through the tree. Everything is revolving. When you are eating an apple, who knows? Your grandfather, your grand-mother, or your great-great-grandfather must be there in the apple; chew well, digest well. Otherwise, the old man will not feel good. Let him become a part of your being again. He has been seeking you through the apple. He has come back again.

Everything is interdependent. So it is not nice, it is not bitter; it is a simple fact. You cannot evaluate it, because nice and bitter are our evaluations, interpretations. And it is not a concept, it is a reality.

"But how is that possible when you urge all of us to be totally selfish?"

Yes, it is only possible if you are totally selfish. If you are totally selfish, you will come to see that if you want to be really happy, you have to make others happy—because life is an interdependence. When I say to be selfish, I am saying to just think about your happiness. But in that happiness much is involved. If you want to be healthy, you have to live with healthy people. If you want to be clean, you have to live in a clean neighborhood. You cannot exist like an island. If you want to be happy you have to spread your happiness all around. It is not possible that all around there is an ocean of misery, and you are like an island, happy—impossible. You can be happy only in a happy world; you can be happy only in happy relationships; you can be beautiful only with beautiful people. So if you are really interested in being beautiful, create beauty all around you.

A man who is really selfish becomes altruistic. To be really
selfish is to go beyond self. To be really selfish is to become a
Buddha, a Jesus. These people are absolutely selfish people because
they think only of bliss. But in thinking of their bliss, they have to
think of others' bliss also. I am absolutely selfish. I have never
thought about anything else but my own self. But in that, from the
back door, enters everything.

I am interested in your happiness, in your bliss. I am interested
to create a community of blissful people. I am interested to create a
garden of beautiful people, because if you are happy and blissful
and beautiful, I will become tremendously blissful and happy.

Bliss increases in sharing. If you don't share your bliss it will die.
If you don't share your ecstasy, soon you will find that your hands
are empty. So when I say be absolutely selfish, I mean: that if you
try to understand what is your self, what your selfishness is, you
will see that everybody is implied, involved. And your involvement
becomes greater and greater and bigger and bigger. A moment
comes when you can see as a fact that the whole is involved.

There is a beautiful story about Buddha.

He reached the ultimate door. The door was opened, but he
would not enter. The doorkeeper said, "Everything is ready, and we
have been waiting for millions of years. Now you have come.
Rarely it happens that a man becomes a Buddha. Enter. Why are
you standing there? And why do you look so sad?" Buddha said,
"How can I enter? Because there are millions of people who are
still struggling on the path. There are millions of people who are
still in misery. I will enter only when everybody else has entered. I
will stand here and wait."

Now, this parable has many meanings. One meaning is that
unless the whole becomes enlightened, how can one become enlightened? Because we are parts of each other, involved in each
other, members of each other. You are in me, I am in you, so how
can I separate myself? It is impossible. The story is tremendously
significant and true. The whole has to become enlightened.

Of course, one can come to a certain understanding, but that
understanding will reveal that others are involved, and the consciousness is one. To be selfish is to dissolve completely into the
total, because only foolish people try to protect themselves. And in
trying to protect themselves they go on destroying themselves.
Jesus says, "Save yourself and you will be lost. Lose yourself. Save
yourself and you will be lost!" He is giving you one of the best

techniques for being selfish: lose yourself, and you gain. You gain by losing yourself. You become happy by spreading happiness all around; you become peaceful by spreading peace all around.

"But how is that possible when you urge all of us to be totally selfish?"

It is possible only if you are totally selfish. Then you will always see the point. If you live in a family, if you are a wife or a husband, you will be able to see that it is in your favor that the husband is happy. It is just selfish that the husband remain happy and singing and delighted, because if he becomes sad, depressed, angry, then you cannot remain happy for long. He will affect you. Everything is infectious. If you want to be happy you would like your children to be dancing and happy, because that is the only way your energy will be dancing. If they are all sad, ill, and sitting in their corners, dull, your energy will immediately fall low. Just watch! When you move with people who are happy, suddenly your sadness disappears—disappears! When you move with people who are sad, suddenly your energy falls low.

Then the mathematics is simple. If you want to be happy, make people happy. If you want to be really enlightened, help people to become enlightened. If you want to be meditative, create a meditative world. That's why Buddha created a great order of sannyasins: an oceanic atmosphere in which people could come and drown themselves.

Just the other night one sannyasin came and he said, "I am feeling very uncomfortable with sannyas, because I feel as if I have become just a part of the herd." Now, this is a very egoistic attitude. Just part of the herd? Everybody wants to be apart, everybody wants to be independent, oneself, alone like a peak, unconnected. This is what the ego-trip is. I give you ochre robes, change your names, and by and by, you are lost in an ocean where you don't exist separately. You start merging yourself with others. Of course, the ego will feel hurt, uncomfortable, uneasy. But the ego is your disease; it has to be dropped. And one should be able to enjoy being a non-entity, being so ordinary, so mixed, that nobody ever comes to know that you are separate, different from others. But the ego has only one idea: how to be separate and different.

I have not told that sannyasin. I wanted to tell him but I thought that maybe it would hurt him—such an egoist who thinks that just being in orange feels very uncomfortable, he has become part of the herd—I wanted to say to him that it is better that you shave half your head, half your moustache, half your beard, so wherever you go you will be separate. And tattoo your forehead, and do things which nobody is doing. You will always feel good and very comfortable. Ego is doing that.

I have heard about one man who wanted to become very famous, who wanted to see his pictures in the newspapers. He shaved half his head, half the moustache, and half the beard, and he walked around the town. Within three days he was the most famous man around the town. All the newspapers had his pictures, and children were running around him and yelling and shouting, and he enjoyed it very much. You can do the same, in the same way.

The ego wants to be separate; and that's why the ego is false, because separation is false. To be together is to be real. All separation is false and illusory, and all togetherness is true and real.

The fifth question:

During the lecture you used the term, 'attain to happiness', and my mind jumped in and said: work more, work harder. But how can I work towards surrender? That feels crazy.

This is from Amida.

She has a great work-oriented mind: work is valuable, play is valueless; and all that has to be achieved, has to be achieved through work. That has become an ingrained habit in her mind. But this has been taught to everybody. The whole world lives according to work ethics. Play is, at the most, tolerated. Work is appreciated.

So even here, when I am talking about surrender, when I am talking about being receptive and feminine, your mind goes on popping. Whenever it finds any support, immediately it pops up and says, "Yes." The very word 'attainment' has started a chain of thoughts within you: attainment?—work, hard work has to be done. Just the word has triggered a certain chain of thoughts, as if the mind was just waiting and watching to jump upon anything which could give it a continuity.

That's how you listen to me. I have to use words, words which are very loaded, words which you have interpreted in different ways, words which have different connotations to you, associations, meanings. I have to use language, and language is a very dangerous thing. Just listening to the word 'attainment', the whole work-oriented mind comes to function. Then you don't listen to me, to what I am saying. I am saying that attainment is possible only when you don't try to attain. Attainment is possible only when all effort to attain is dropped, because that which you are trying to attain is already there. It cannot be attained. The very effort to attain it will continue to create barriers between you and your reality. But the mind goes on watching, and is always ready to find some support for itself.

Let me tell you one anecdote.

The policeman in a small village had been there some twenty years and he was not very popular with the residents. Far from being the local village bobby who was as much a member of the populus as the local butcher or the local postman, he had always seen himself as the sheriff in a Western film, and treated even the most minor infringement as if it were a case for New Scotland Yard. It was his proud boast that every resident of the village had received a summons as a result of his devotion to duty. As the time approached when he would be replaced by a police car which would cover no less than six villages, including the one which he had come to regard as his own, he suddenly realized that he had never had a case against the local vicar. And his pride could not allow him to retire without bringing this man to justice. His task appeared hopeless. But as he watched the vicar cycling around the village, one day he hit upon a master plan. Positioning himself at the bottom of the only hill in the village, he waited for the vicar to cycle down. When the vicar was about a yard away, the constable stepped in front of him, thinking to himself, "He will run over my foot. It will hurt, but I will get him for not having adequate brakes." The vicar's reflexes however, enabled him to stop his bicycle an eighth of an inch in front of the policeman's boots. The constable reluctantly admitted defeat and said, "I thought I had you that time, vicar."

The vicar said, "Oh yes, but God was with me."

"Got you!" said the policeman. "Two on a bike!"

That's how the mind goes on—watching. Any excuse: rational, irrational; any excuse, even any absurdity, and the mind immediately jumps and tries to continue in the old pattern. I am saying so many things to you, and of course, I have to use language. Be alert, be alert of this tricky mind which is just hiding there behind you, and just waiting for something which can be an excuse for its being strengthened more.

Work is good; but work as work is ugly, not good. Work is good if
it is also a play. Work is good if it has an intrinsic value; you paint
because you love to paint, because you enjoy painting. Of course, if
the painting is sold and you receive some money, that is secondary,
that is irrelevant, that is not the point. If you get the money, good;
if you don't get the money, you are not missing anything, because
you were so delighted while painting. You are almost rewarded.
More than your effort, you have been rewarded. If the painting can
be sold that is a plus reward: God is being too kind to you. But as
far as your reward is concerned, you have already got it. When you
paint your painting, when you write your poem, when you work in
the garden and perspire in the sun, you have got your reward.

Work as play, work as enjoyment, work as worship—then it is
beautiful; it has a grace to it. Work as an economic activity is ugly.
Then you become a part of the market-place. Then you are thinking
only in terms of what you are going to get out of it. Then you are
never here-now. Then you are always in the result, and the result is
in the future. Never be result-oriented—that is the misery of the
human mind—be present-oriented. And you are not going to get
your innermost being through work. You are going to get it by
being present, by being aware. So use your work also as a situation.

But what happens? You listen to me: you go on noting down
inside your mind what I am saying. You don't really listen to me.
You go on collecting cues. You don't collect understanding. You
collect cues, and that's what creates problems.

Let me tell you another anecdote.

In the old days, the doctor took his assistant with him to the
bedside of the patient. The Irish priest's face was red, and his
temperature was high. The doctor slapped him on the back. "Get
up, and eat some corned beef and cabbage," he told him. The next
day the Irishman was back at work. The apprentice made a note:
red face, high temperature—corned beef and cabbage.

Shortly afterwards, in the absence of the doctor, the young man
was himself called to the bedside of a German patient whose face
was red and who had a high temperature. The apprentice pre-
scribed corned beef and cabbage. The very next day they notified
the apprentice that the German was dead. He then entered the
following in his notebook: corned beef and cabbage—good for
Irishmen, kills Germans.

This is what you are doing with me—collecting cues. Just try to
understand what I am saying. Don't collect cues. Just watch me,
what I am doing here. What is transpiring between me and you

here, right in this moment; what energy exchange is happening between you and me right this moment: watch it, feel it, and let it be dissolved into your being. Don't take notes, otherwise you will be always in trouble.

The last question:

> . . . and very serious, Please don't take it as a joke. Chitananda has asked,

> *By the way, you are the only non-neurotic person around. Why don't you have children? Do enlightened persons have children sometimes?*

I never thought about it.

You may not learn anything from my answers, but I go on learning from your questions: a very good idea. I will remember it. But there is a practical problem: it is very difficult to find a non-neurotic woman.

First, it is difficult to find a non-neurotic person, and then a woman?—almost impossible. The difficulty is multiplied.

Let me tell you one anecdote.

A very wealthy city financier was a wizard on the stock exchange but was very lousy on the golf course. He was in the habit of taking out his bad temper on his caddy, and one morning, after a particularly bad round, he shouted, "You must be just about the worst caddy in the world!" "Oh, no sir," replied the caddy, "that would be too much of a coincidence!"

The worst golfer and the worst caddy in the world?—that would be too much of a coincidence.

To find a non-neurotic woman would be too much of a coincidence. It has not happened before, and I don't think it can happen. Never has it been known that any enlightened man had any children. Yes, you may have heard that Buddha had a son, but that happened before he became enlightened.

Mahavir had a daughter, but that too happened before he became enlightened. Gurdjieff had many children from many women, but that too happened before he became enlightened. And you must be well aware that those children, even Buddha's son Rahul, did not prove much of a Buddha's son. Mahavir's daughter has not proved in any way a Mahavir's daughter; she proved ordinary. She was so ordinary that one of the sects of Jainas believes that this is just a myth: Mahavir never got married and he never had any children. The daughter was so ordinary, almost as if she was not. Have you ever heard of any enlightened person's son or daughter becoming enlightened? The coincidence is too much of a coincidence.

And there is something else involved. First, a non-neurotic person finding a non-neurotic woman, and then both together finding a non-neurotic soul to be born. The problem is very complicated because you seek a woman only because you are neurotic. Because you have not met with your inner woman yet, you seek a woman. You seek a man because you have not met with your inner man yet. Because you are not a complete whole inside, you go out.

First, the moment you become a whole inside—that's the meaning of being a holy person, a person who is whole—then you don't seek outside. There is no need. You also don't escape. If a woman comes along, you don't run away and you don't report to the police that a woman is coming along. That too is good. If a woman comes along, perfectly good. If she goes away, that too is perfectly good.

And you give birth to children; that too out of neurosis—because you always want occupation, somewhere to be occupied. Your basic occupation is with the future, and children make the future available to you. Through them, your ambitions will be able to move. When you are gone, your children will be here. When you were trying to become a prime minister and you could not, your children will become. You will prepare them and the continuity will be there.

When one dies, and if one does not leave any children behind, one feels at a dead-end, a cul-de-sac. But when you leave children behind you feel a sort of immortality through them: "That's okay; I am dying, nothing to worry about. But a part of me will be living through my child." People are much too interested in children because they are much too afraid of death. Children give you a false notion of immortality, a continuity of some sort. A non-neurotic person is not interested in children, is not interested in any sort of continuity. He has found the eternal, and he is not worried about death.

A few anecdotes about why it is so impossible to find a non-neurotic woman . . . I will not comment; I will simply read a few anecdotes.

Mrs. Cohen had come into some money and asked an interior

decorator to re-do her house. Mr. Jones asked, "Certainly Mrs. Cohen, I will be glad to help. Can you give me some idea of your taste? Do you like modern decor?"

"No."

"Swedish style?"

"No."

"Italian provincial?"

"No."

"Moorish? Spanish?"

"No."

"Well you know, Mrs. Cohen, you really must give me some idea of your taste, otherwise I will not even be able to get started. What is it exactly that you have in mind?"

"Decor, schmecor. What I want is that when my friends come to visit, they will take one look and drop dead!"

The second: The young couple was engaged in a most affectionate embrace when there came the sound of a key in the front door. The young lady broke away at once, eyes wide with alarm. "Heavens!" she cried, "it is my husband. Quick, jump out of the window!"

The young man, equally alarmed, made a step toward the window, then demurred. "I can't! We are on the thirteenth floor!"

"For heaven's sake!" cried the young lady in exasperation. "Is this a time to be superstitious?"

Third: The wife came home wearing a new hat. "Where did you get that hat?" her husband asked.

"At a clearance sale."

"No wonder they wanted to clear it out," he said. "It makes you look like an idiot."

"I know it."

"Then why in the world did you buy it?" he demanded.

"I will tell you," she said. "When I put it on and looked at myself in the mirror, I looked too stupid to argue with the clerk."

The fourth: Mulla Nasrudin was telling me that marriage is the process of finding out what kind of man your wife would have preferred. "My wife said to me this morning, 'If you really loved me, you would have married someone else.' I assured her that I was very happy being married to her, and said, 'If I could change places with Richard Burton, I would not do it.' She said, 'I know you wouldn't. You never do anything to please me.'"

CHAPTER FIVE
May 5, 1976

THIS IS IT!

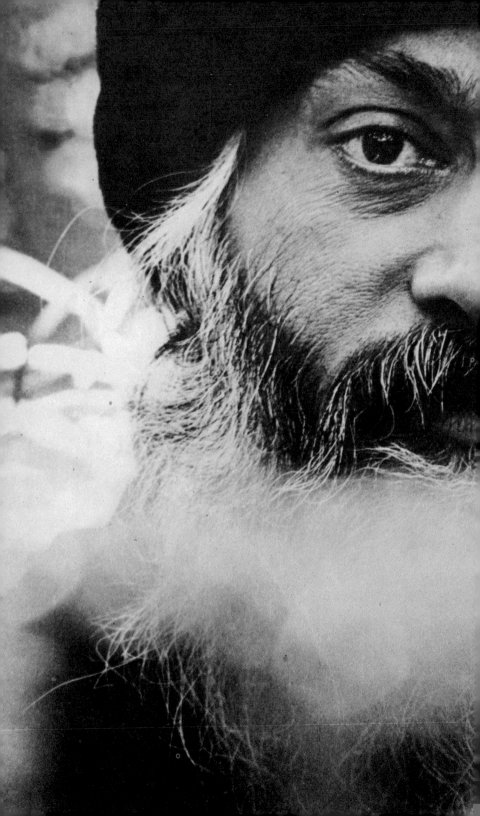

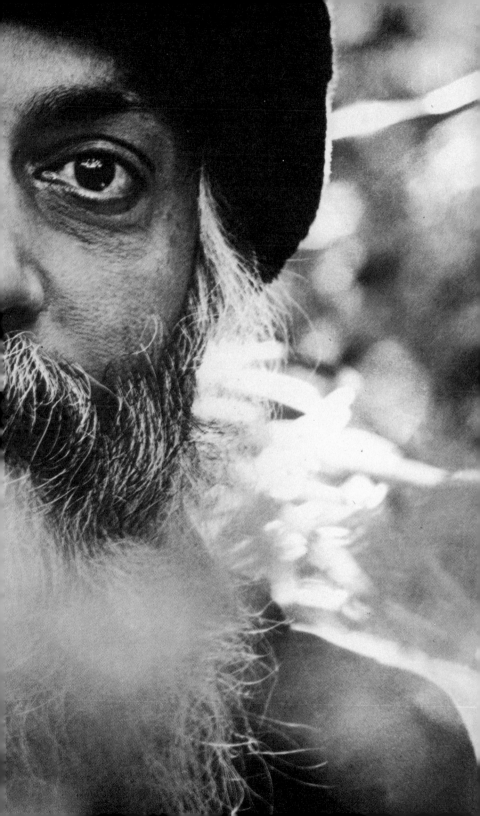

11

Being bound together as cause-effect, the effects disappear with the disappearance of causes.

हेतुफलाश्रयालम्बनैः संगृहीतत्वादेषामभावे तदभावः ॥ ११ ॥

12

Past and future exist in the present, but they are not experienced in the present because they are on different planes.

अतीतानागतं स्वरूपतोऽस्त्यध्वभेदाद्धर्माणाम् ॥ १२ ॥

13

Whether manifest or unmanifest, the past, the present and the future are of the nature of gunas: stability, action and inertia.

ते व्यक्तसूक्ष्मा गुणात्मानः ॥ १३ ॥

14

The essence of any object consists in the uniqueness of the proportions of the three gunas.

परिणामैकत्वाद्वस्तुतत्त्वम् ॥ १४ ॥

15

The same object is seen in different ways by different minds.

वस्तुसाम्ये चित्तभेदात्तयोर्विभक्तः पन्थाः ॥ १५ ॥

16

An object is not dependent on one mind.

न चैकचित्ततन्त्रं वस्तु तदप्रमाणकं तदा किं स्यात् ॥ १६ ॥

17

An object is known or unknown depending on whether the mind is colored by it or not.

तदुपरागापेक्षित्वाच्चित्तस्य वस्तु ज्ञाताज्ञातम् ॥ १७ ॥

The first sutra:

Being bound together as cause-effect, the effects
disappear with the disappearance of causes.

AVIDYA, ignorance of one's own being, is the basic cause of
the world. Once avidya, the ignorance of one's own being,
disappears, the world also disappears—not the world of
objects, but the world of desires; not the world that is
outside you, but the world that you have been constantly projecting
from the inside. The world of your dreams, illusions, projections,
immediately disappears the moment ignorance disappears within
you.

This has to be understood: ignorance is not simply lack of
knowledge, so you can go on gathering knowledge but ignorance
will not disappear that way. You can become very knowledgeable,
but still you will remain ignorant. In fact, knowledge functions as a
protection for ignorance. Ignorance is not destroyed by knowledge.
On the contrary, it is protected by it. The urge to collect knowledge,
accumulate knowledge, is nothing but to hide one's own ignorance.
The more you know, the more you think that now you are no longer
ignorant.

There is a saying in Tibet: Blessed are they who are ignorant, for
they are happy in thinking that they know everything.

Trying to know everything is not going to help; it is missing the
whole point. Trying to know one's self is enough. If you can know
your own being you have known all because you participate with
the whole, your nature is of the whole.

You are just like a drop of water. If you know the drop·of water
totally, you have known all the oceans, past, present and future. In
a single drop of water the whole nature of the ocean is present.

A man who is after knowledge continuously forgets himself and
goes on accumulating information. He may come to know much,
but still he will remain ignorant. So ignorance is not against
knowledge; knowledge is not the antidote for ignorance. Then what
is the antidote for ignorance? Yoga says: awareness; not knowledge,
but knowing; not focusing yourself outside, but focusing on the very
faculty of knowing.

When a child is in the mother's womb, he is completely asleep. The first months in the mother's womb are of deep sleep, what yoga calls *sushupti*—sleep without any dreams. Then, by the end of the sixth or seventh month, the child starts a little dreaming. The sleep is disturbed; it is no more absolute. Something happens outside, a noise, and the child's sleep is disturbed. Vibrations reach him, and in his deep sleep a distraction arrives and he starts dreaming. The first ripples of dream arise. Dreamless sleep is the first state of consciousness.

The second state is: sleep plus dream. In the second state sleep remains, but a new faculty starts functioning: the faculty of dreaming. Then, when the child is born a third faculty arises, what we ordinarily call the state of waking. It is not really the state of waking, but a new faculty starts functioning and that faculty is of thought. The child starts thinking.

The first state was dreamless sleep: the second state was sleep plus dreaming; the third state is sleep, plus dreaming, plus thinking, but sleep still remains. Sleep has not been completely broken. You remain asleep in your thinking also. Your thinking is nothing but another way of dreaming; the sleep is not disturbed. These are the ordinary states. Rarely does a man reach higher than this third stage, of thinking. And that is the goal of yoga: to reach to a state of pure awareness, as pure as the first state is. The first state is of pure sleep, and the last state is of pure awakening, pure awareness. Once your awareness is as pure as your deep sleep, you have become a Buddha, you have attained, you have come home.

= DREAMLESS SLEEP

Patanjali says: *samadhi*, the ultimate state of awareness, is just like sleep, with one difference. It is as calm and quiet as sleep, as silent, undisturbed as sleep, as integrated and blissful as sleep, with one difference: it is fully alert. These are the points of evolution. Ordinarily, we remain at the third. Deep down sleep continues, on top of it a layer of dreaming, on top of it another layer of thinking—but the sleep is not broken. And you can observe it; it is not a theory. You can observe the facticity of it.

At any moment you close your eyes, first you will see thoughts, a layer of thinking all around you, thoughts vibrating—one coming, another going—a crowd, a traffic. Remain silent for a few seconds, and suddenly you will see that thinking is no longer there but dreaming has started. You are dreaming that you have become the president of a country, or you have found a brick of gold on the road, or you have found a beautiful woman or a man, and suddenly you start projecting; dreams start functioning. If you continue dreaming for a long time, one moment will come when you will fall asleep—thinking, dreaming, sleep, and from sleep again to dreaming and thinking. This is how your whole life revolves. Real awareness is not known yet, and that real awareness is what Patanjali says will destroy ignorance—not knowledge, but awareness. We collect knowledge just to befool ourselves and others.

I have heard: In a small school it happened that a school inspector said to the class, "Who knocked down the walls of Jericho?" And one of the pupils, a lad called Billy Green, replied promptly, "Please sir, it was not me." The inspector was amazed at this show of ignorance and brought the matter up in the headmaster's study at the end of the visit. "Do you know," he said, "I asked the class, 'Who knocked down the walls of Jericho,' and young Billy Green said it was not him!" The headmaster said, "Billy Green? Oh well . . . I must say that I have always found the lad to be honest and trustworthy, and if he says that it was not him, then it was not him."

The inspector left the school without further comment, but lost no time in reporting the full sequence of events to the Ministry of Education in a written report. In due course, he received the following reply: "Dear sir, Reference: The Walls of Jericho; this is a matter for the Ministry of Works, and your letter has been sent to them for their attention."

But nobody wants to recognize a simple fact, that they don't know. Everybody tries; whatsoever the question, everybody tries the answer. You should catch yourself red-handed many times if you try. Somebody asks something, somebody talks about something you don't know, but you start commenting, advising, saying something or other so that you are not caught ignorant, so nobody thinks that you are ignorant. But the first beginning of awareness starts with the recognition that you are ignorant. Ignorance can be destroyed, but not without recognizing it.

When P. D. Ouspensky, the great disciple of George Gurdjieff, met his Master for the first time, he was already a very famous, well known man in the world. Gurdjieff was unknown, Ouspensky was known very much already. He had already written one of the best books written in this century, *Tertium Organum*. It is really a bold attempt. In fact, in this century no other man has tried such a bold speculation. With courage, Ouspensky has described his book as the third canon of thought: *tertium organum*. The first was written by Aristotle; the second was written by Bacon. And he said, "I write the third canon of thought." He said, "The first and the second are nothing before the third. The third existed before the first." It was really a bold attempt, and not just egoistic. The claim was almost true.

When Ouspensky went to Gurdjieff, Gurdjieff looked at him. He could see the knowledgeable man who knew much, who knew that others also knew that he knew much—the subtle ego. Gurdjieff gave him a paper, a sheet of paper, and told him to go to a room on the side and write down on one side whatsoever he knew, and on the other side whatsoever he did not know. Because the work could start only when he was clear about what he knew and what he did not know. Gurdjieff said, "Remember, whatsoever you write that you know, I will accept, and we will never talk about it again. It is finished; you know. Whatsoever you write that you don't know, we will work on it." And the first thing Gurdjieff said was to know what you know and what you don't know.

Ouspensky went into the room. He started thinking of what he knew for the first time in his life, and he could not write a single thing on the paper. He tried God, self, the world, mind, aware- ness—what did he know? For the first time the question was asked authentically. He knew many things about God, and he knew many things about the soul, and he knew many things about awareness, but he did not really know a thing about God. It was all informa- tion; it was not his experience. And unless something is your experience how can you say you know it?

You may know about love, but that is not knowledge really. You have to pass through love, you have to pass through the fire of love. You have to burn, you have to survive the challenge, and when you come out of love you are totally different, different from the man who had gone in. Love transforms. Information never transforms you. Information goes on becoming an addition: whatsoever you are, it goes on adding to it. It becomes like a treasure to you but you remain the same. Experience changes you. Real knowledge is not an accumulation, it is a transformation, a mutation—the old dies and the new is born. It is hard. . . .

Ouspensky tried as hard as possible to find at least a few things, because it was so much against his ego not to write anything. He could not even write, "I know myself." If you have not known the basic entity, yourself, then what else can you know? It was a cold night and he started perspiring. Just a moment before he was shivering with cold. His whole being was at stake. He started feeling dizzy, as if he would fall into a swoon or a fit. Long hours passed, then Gurdjieff knocked at the door and said, "Have you done anything?" And Gurdjieff could see that the man had changed. Just keeping that blank sheet of paper in his hand, sitting there—it had been a great meditation, a zazen. He gave the empty, blank paper to Gurdjieff and said, "I don't know anything. I am absolutely ignorant. Accept me as your disciple." Gurdjieff said, "You are ready then . . . to recognize that one is ignorant is the first step towards wisdom."

Being bound together as cause-effect, the effects
disappear with the disappearance of causes.

Patanjali says that you are immoral, but that is an effect. You are greedy, but that is an effect. You feel anger; that is an effect. Find out the cause. Don't go on fighting with the effects because that is not going to help. You can fight with your greed, and it will appear again from somewhere else. You can fight with your anger; it will be repressed and will explode somewhere again. Effects cannot be destroyed by fighting with effects. That's why yoga is not a system of morality, it is a system of awareness. The real cause has to be found. If you go on cutting and pruning the leaves of a tree it is not going to affect the tree. New leaves will come up. You will have to seek out the roots, the very cause. If you want to destroy the tree you will have to destroy the roots. With the roots destroyed, the tree will disappear. But you can go on cutting the branches; it is not going to destroy the tree. In fact, wherever you cut one branch, three will come up. Prune a tree and it becomes denser and thicker. Cut the roots and the tree disappears.

Yoga says: morality goes on fighting with the effects.

You are greedy, you try to be non-greedy, but what happens? You can be non-greedy only if your greed can be diverted towards non-greed. If somebody says that if you become non-greedy you will go to heaven, and if you remain greedy you will go to hell, now what is he doing? He is giving you a new object for your greed. He is saying, "Become non-greedy; you will attain to paradise and you will be happy there forever and ever." Now, a greedy person will start thinking how to practice non-greed so he can reach to heaven.

You are afraid; fear is there. How to get rid of fear? You can be made more afraid, and so much fear can be created about fear that you start repressing it. But that is not going to make you fearless; you will simply become more afraid. A new fear will arise, the fear of fear.

You are angry. It is simple for you to become angry, and very difficult to resist the temptation. Now something can be done. Why do you become angry? Whenever your ego is hurt, you become angry. Now it can be taught to you that a man who is controlled is respected in society. A man who does not show his anger so easily is thought to be a great man. Then your ego is being enhanced: become more disciplined and controlled, and don't be so easily tempted to become angry. Your ego is not destroyed; rather, it is strengthened. The disease may change its form, name, but the disease will remain. Remember this: yoga is not a system of morality because it doesn't bother about effects. That's why there is no such thing as ten commandments.

People go on teaching each other without knowing the basic cause. And unless the basic cause is known, nothing can be done; the human personality remains the same; maybe a little modified here and there, polished here and there.

I have heard: A Polish man went to the eye hospital for an eye test. Seated in front of the chart, the doctor asked him to read through the lines one at a time. As the man got to the bottom line which read: C S V E N C J W, he hesitated. The doctor said, "Don't look so worried. If you can't read it, just try your best." The Polish man said, "Read it? I know the fellow personally!"

It is so hard to accept that you don't know, that you don't know why you are egoistic. You don't know why you get so easily angry. You don't know why greed is there. You don't know why lust is there, why fear is there. Without knowing the cause, you start fighting with the effects. You assume that you know. Many people come to me and they say, "Somehow, we would like to get rid of anger." I ask them, "Do you know the cause?" They shrug their shoulders. They say, "Just, anger is there, and I get very easily angry and it disturbs me, disturbs my relationship, makes me more tense, creates anxiety, repentance, guilt." But these are all effects.

Why, in the first place, does anger arise?—nobody asks. And this is the beauty of it: if you ask about the cause, if you enquire about the cause, you will be surprised to find out that the cause is one. There are millions of effects but the cause is one, the root is one. Anger, greed, ego, lust, fear, hatred, jealousy, envy, violence: whatsoever the effect, the cause is one. And the cause is: that you are not aware enough. You can control anger, but that will not help you. It will be just controlling the disease within you, holding it in. It will not make you healthy. It may even make you more unhealthy. You can see—a person who gets easily angry is never very dangerous. You can be certain that he will never commit any murder. He will never accumulate enough anger to become a murderer. Every day he catharts. Easily, with any provocation, he gets angry. That means that his steam no longer accumulates in him. He has a leaking system. Whenever there is too much steam, he lets it go. A man who is very much controlled is a dangerous man. He goes on holding in steam; his energies become pent-up, dammed. One day or other the energies will prove more than his control. Then he will explode, then he will do something really grave. A man who easily gets angry, easily cools also.

I have heard: "I'm sorry sir," said the clerk, "but I'm giving in my notice."

"But why?" asked his boss in surprise.

"Well sir, to tell you the truth, I can't stand your foul temper."

"Oh, come now," pleaded the boss. "I know I can be a bit grumpy at times, but you must admit that no sooner is my temper on than it is off."

"That's true sir, but also, as soon as it is off, it is on again."

But this type of man can never be a murderer. He never accumulates that much steam. People who simply get emotional are good people. They may not be very controlled, they can cry and weep and laugh, but they are good people. To be with them is better than to be with a religious man—moralistic, puritan, very collected, controlled. He's dangerous.

Just a few days ago a young man had been in Teertha's encounter group. He had taken training for many years in aikido. Now aikido, judo, karate, and all methods of ju-jitsu are disciplines of control. You have to control yourself so much that a person becomes almost a statue, so controlled you cannot provoke him. And this man took part in the encounter group.

Now, the philosophy of an encounter group is totally different. It is to bring out whatsoever is inside you. Never accumulate it. Cathart, let it go, act it out. Encounter and aikido are totally diametrically opposite things. Aikido says: control—because the training of aikido is the training for a warrior. All the Japanese trainings are to make you a great warrior, and certainly they have developed methods which are tremendously dangerous. But they were meant to be so because the Japanese are very small people. Their height is very small, and they had to fight with people who were bigger than them. They had to create devices in which they could prove themselves stronger than the bigger people, stronger people, and they really found devices. The one device is to control every energy in you. It becomes a pooled-up thing. So the Japanese, the Chinese, they have lived with much control, discipline. They are dangerous. Once they attack you they will not leave you alive. Ordinarily, they will not attack you, but once they attack you, you can be certain that they will kill you.

Now this man who had been deeply in aikido was in the encounter group, and Teertha must have been insisting for him to bring things out, and he would not. His whole training—he told me later on—"My whole training is to remain controlled." Now one girl participant in the group started hitting him. She was bringing her anger out, and he remained like a statue because his whole training is to not act out. He remained like a Buddha; not actually a Buddha, because a Buddha remains alert, not controlled. On the surface, both may look the same. A man who is controlled and a man who is aware may look the same, but deep inside they are totally different. Their energy is qualitatively different.

He became more and more angry inside, and also more and more controlled because his whole training was at stake. Then he threw a pillow at the girl, and even a pillow thrown by a man of aikido can be dangerous. He can hit you at such a delicate point, with such force, that even death can occur with a pillow. That is the whole training—one takes years—a small hit, but at the very delicate points.

The Japanese have worked out where to hit very slightly, and the person is gone. Just with a single finger they can defeat the enemy. They have found the delicate points to hit, and how to hit, and when to hit.

But then, he himself became afraid, afraid that he could kill the girl. He became so afraid that he escaped from the group and he came to me and complained. He said, "This type of group should not be allowed in the ashram. Someday, somebody may murder somebody." He's right, because the murderer in him is there. His fear is right; it is right about himself. He can be a murderer. In fact, trainings like that are trainings to make you a murderer of man, to make you a warrior.

Remember, if you control anger, greed, and things like that, they go on accumulating in the basement of your being—and you are sitting on a volcano. Yoga has nothing to do with repression. The belief of yoga is in awareness.

Being bound together as cause-effect, the effects disappear with the disappearance of causes.

Find out the cause, and the cause is one. And things become simple, because you are not to fight with so many effects. You simply cut one root, the main root, and a whole tree of a thousand and one branches simply disappears, withers away. Become more aware.

Out of sleep arises the dream state; dreams start floating. Have you seen, sometimes in a dream you dream that you are awake? Exactly the same is happening: in thinking, you think you are awake. As in a dream you can dream you are awake, in thinking you can think you are awake—but you are not. Real awakening happens only when all thoughts have disappeared—there is no cloud inside you, not a single thought floating, just pure you. It is just a purity, a clarity of perception; just a vision with no object in your vision, the whole sky empty. If you look at anything, no word arises in you. You see a rose flower: not even this much arises in you, that "This is a beautiful flower." You simply see the rose there, you here, and between you two, no verbalization. In that silence, for the first time you know what being aware is, what is this state of wakefulness—and that cuts the root. Now try it in many ways.

One way is: when you get angry try to be aware. Suddenly, you will see that either you can be angry or you can be aware; you cannot be both together. When sexuality arises try to be aware. Suddenly, you will see that either you can be aware or you can be sexual; you cannot be both together. That will help you to see the fact: that awareness is the antidote, not control. If you become more and more aware, energy starts moving in a totally different dimension. The same energy that was moving in anger, in greed, in sex, is freed, starts moving like a pillar of light inside you. And that awareness is the highest state of human evolution. A man becomes a God when he is aware. Unless you attain to that, your life has been a wastage. We live as if we are drunk.

Let me tell you a few anecdotes.

After a wild night in Old Mexico, the tourist woke up with a raging hangover and only a dim memory of the night before. Beside him in the bed lay a filthy, ugly, wrinkled and toothless hag. Retching with disgust, he ran to the bathroom, where he bumped into a pretty, young Mexican girl. "Hey, was I drunk last night?" he asked her. "I think you must have been," came the reply. "Otherwise you would not have married my mother."

Whatsoever you have done up to now, one day, suddenly you will see that all has gone wrong. Whosoever you are married to, whatsoever your life has been motivated by up to now, whatsoever your desire has been up to now, one day you will become aware and see that it has always been as if you have been drunk.

John Smith was a notorious tippler. One night, after an evening on the town, he was taking a short-cut home through a cemetery when he tripped over a gravestone and fell flat on his face. He did not regain consciousness until the next morning, and the first thing he saw when he opened his eyes was the gravestone above his head. Now, John Smith is a common name, and the grave he was lying on happened to belong to another man with the same name. As the words 'Sacred to the Memory of John Smith' came into focus, he muttered to himself, "Well, that's me alright, but I don't remember a damned thing about the funeral!"

When a person starts meditating, he is coming out of a long drunkenness of many lives. For the first time, one cannot even believe how one has lived up to now. It seems like a nightmare— horrible. That's why people don't even try to be aware, because the first glimpse of awareness is going to scatter, to destroy their whole life that they had been thinking had any meaning up to now. Their whole life is going to become meaningless, insignificant. The fear of awareness is the fear that it may prove your whole life wrong. That's why only very courageous people try to meditate, try to become aware. Otherwise, people just go on moving in the same vicious circle of the same desires, and the same dreams, and the same thoughts; and they come again and again back to life, and again die—from the cradle to the grave. . . .

Just start thinking a little, contemplate about what you have been doing: repeating a few unconscious desires, repeating something which never gives you any blissfulness, which always frustrates you. Still you go on as if you are hypnotized. In fact, that's what yoga says: that we are in a deep hypnosis. Nobody else has hypnotized us, we are hypnotized by our own minds; but we live in a hypnosis.

I have heard: As the drunk staggered homeward, he was wracking his brains for a means of concealing his condition from his wife. Finally he thought of a bright idea: he could go in and pick up a book. "After all," he thought, "who ever heard of a drunk reading a book?" Putting his plan into action, he let himself into his house, walked straight into the lounge and sat down. A minute later, his wife came stamping down the stairs and peered round the door. "What do you think you're doing?" she asked. "Just reading, dear," replied the drunk. "You're blind drunk again, you alcoholic idiot," ranted his wife. "Now close that suitcase and come to bed."

Whatsoever you are doing in your unconscious state, *whatsoever* it is, I say unconditionally, is going to be idiotic. You also feel that sometimes, but again and again you drop the subject. You don't remember it for too long because that seems to be too much of a risk.

You love a woman: if you became aware, the love might disappear because your love might be just a hypnosis, as it is ordinarily. You are ambitious, you are trying to reach to the capital to become a president or a prime minister: now you will be afraid of becoming aware, because if you become aware suddenly the whole thing will look stupid, and you have staked your whole life for it.

Just the other day I saw a picture of Senator Humphrey crying, because he had been trying for his whole life to become the President of America, and this was his last chance, and there seemed to be no possibility. So, standing before his admirers he started weeping. Tears came to his eyes and he said, "Now I am old, and this seems to be my last chance; I will never be standing again for President." Crying like a small child . . . your politicians are just small children playing and fighting with each other.

If you become aware, you may suddenly see the whole nonsense of your efforts. You may stop, and that 'somewhere' deep inside you is always felt. You are after money. . . .

Once it happened: A very rich man used to come to listen to me. Suddenly he stopped. After many months I suddenly met him on a morning walk. I asked him, "Where have you been? You have disappeared suddenly?" He said, "Not suddenly; but I became, by and by, afraid. I will come to listen to you, but now is not the time. I am young, and listening to you, by and by, I was getting less and less ambitious. Now that will be dangerous. I have to attain my ambitions first. In my later years, when I have become old, then I will meditate, but this is not for me now. First I had come to you just out of curiosity, but by and by, I was getting caught in it. I stopped myself. It was difficult to stop, but I am a man of will-power."

You cannot become aware because you have many investments in your foolishness, in your ignorance, in your unawareness. In this sleep, in this slumber, you have invested your life, and many things. Now, the first ray of awareness, and you will feel that your whole life has been a wastage. You are still not courageous. That's why people go on changing effects, because then there is no danger. And they never touch the root.

Once it happened: I was travelling with Mulla Nasrudin. Suddenly he became aware that he had lost his ticket. He looked in all his pockets: in the coat, in the shirt, in the pants—but I was watching. He was not looking in one of his pockets. So I told him, "You are looking in every pocket, in the suitcase, in the bag and everything. Why don't you look in this pocket?" He said, "I am afraid. If the ticket is not there I will drop dead. I am leaving it so that the hope remains that if it is not anywhere, at least that pocket is still there; maybe it is there? If I look into it and it is not there, I will drop dead."

You know where to look, but still you are afraid. Then you go on looking in other places just to remain occupied. You go on looking in money, in power, in prestige, in this and that, but never inside you, never in your inner being. You are afraid; it seems that if you look there and nothing is found you will drop dead. But those who have looked there have always found. Not a single exception has ever happened of one who has gone within and has not found the treasure. This is one of the most universal facts. Even scientific facts are not so universal; this fact is without any exception. Whenever, in any country, in any century, any woman or any man have looked into themselves, they have found the treasure. But one has to look, and for that a great daring is needed. You have arranged your world outside of yourself. Your love, your power, your money, your fame, your name: all are outside you. One who wants to go in will have to leave these things, will have to close his eyes; and one clings to the very end.

Life goes on frustrating you; that's a blessing. Life goes on frustrating you again and again. Life is saying, "Go within." All frustrations are simply indications that you are looking in a wrong direction. Fulfillment is possible only in a right direction. Life frustrates you because life is a tremendous blessing. If you are satisfied outside you will be lost forever; then you will never look within. But in spite of all the frustrations you go on hoping.

I have heard about a man: "Why did you quit your last job?" "Well, the boss said I was sacked, but I did not take any notice. He was always saying that. So I went in the next day and all my things had been cleared out of my office. Then I went in the day after and my name plate had been taken off the door, and the following day I found someone else sitting in my chair. 'This is too much!' I thought to myself; so I resigned."

But even that is not too much to you. Every day you are sacked, every day you are fired, every day you are frustrated, every moment. Whatsoever arrangements you make are destroyed every

moment, whatsoever you propose is disposed. All your hopes simply prove hopeless, and all your dreams turn into dust and leave a
very bitter taste in the mouth. You feel continuously nauseous, but
still you go on clinging: some day, maybe, from somewhere, your
dreams may be fulfilled. This is how you go on hanging on to the
very illusory world of your projections. Unless you become alert
and see the hopelessness of your hopes, unless you drop all hoping
you will not turn in, and you will not be able to destroy the cause.

*Past and future exist in the present, but they are not
experienced in the present because they are on
different planes.*

Yoga believes in eternity, not in time. Yoga says: all always
is—the past is still there, hidden in the present, and the future is
also there, hidden in the present—because the past cannot simply
disappear and the future cannot simply appear out of nothingness.
Past, present, future, all are here-now. For us they are divided
because we cannot see the totality. We have very small slits of eyes,
senses, to look at reality. We divide.

If our consciousness is pure and there is no cloud in it, we will
see eternity as it is. There will be no past and there will be no
future. There will only be this moment, eternally this moment.

A great Zen Master, Bokuju, was dying, and his disciples
gathered. The chief disciple asked, "Master, you are leaving us.
People will ask us what your message was, after you are gone.
Though you have been teaching us always and always, you have
taught so many things, and we are ignorant people; it will be
difficult for us to condense your message. So please, before you
leave, give your very essence just in a single sentence." Bokuju
opened his eyes and said loudly, "This is it!" closed his eyes and
died. Now after him, for centuries, people have been asking what he
meant: This is it? He had said everything.

This . . . is . . . it . . .

He had given the whole message: this moment is all there is.
This moment—the whole past, the whole present, the whole future,
is involved in this moment. But you cannot see it in its totality
because your mind is so clouded, so dusty with thought, dream,
sleep; so much hypnosis, desire, motive. You cannot see. You are
not total, your vision is not total. "Once the vision is total,"
Patanjali says, "past and future exist in the present, but they are
not experienced in the present because they are on different
planes." The past has moved on a different plane. It has become

your unconscious, and into your unconscious you cannot move, so
you cannot know your past. The future exists on a different plane: it
exists in your superconscious. But because you cannot move in your
superconscious you cannot know your future. You are closed in
your small consciousness, very fragmentary. You are just like the
tip of an iceberg: much is hidden deep, just beneath you, and much
is hidden just above you. Just below, and above, and the whole
reality surrounds you, but you are clinging to a very small consciousness. Make this consciousness greater and bigger.

That's what meditation is all about—how to make your consciousness bigger, how to make your consciousness infinite. You
will only be able to know that much reality; in the same proportion
will you be able to know the reality as you have consciousness. If
you have infinite consciousness you will know the infinite; if you
have momentary consciousness you will know the moment. On
your consciousness depends everything.

Whether manifest or unmanifest, the past, the
present, and the future are of the nature of the three
gunas: stability, action and inertia.

We have talked in the past about the three gunas: *sattva* means
stability, *rajas* means action, and *tamas* means inertia. Patanjali
now joins past, present, and future with the three gunas. For
Patanjali, everything in life and existence is somehow joined with
the three gunas, the three attributes of existence. That is Patanjali's
trinity. Everything consists of three things. Stability; the past is
stability. That's why you cannot change your past; it has become
almost stable. Now you cannot change it. There is no way to change
it. It has become permanent. The present is action, rajas. The
present is a continuous process, movement. Present is dynamic and
future is inertia. It is still in the seed, fast asleep. In the seed the
tree is asleep, is in inertia.

The future is the potential, the past is the actual, and the present
is the movement of the potential towards the actual. The past is
that which has happened, the future is that which is going to
happen, and the present is the passage between the two. Present is
the passage of the future to become past, for the seed to become the
tree.

The essence of any object consists in the uniqueness
of the proportions of the three gunas.

Now physicists say that the electron, neutron, and proton are the basic elements, and everything is made of these. Everything is made of these three: the positive, the neutral and the negative. That is exactly the meaning of sattva, rajas, and tamas: the positive, the neutral, and the negative—and everything is made of these three. Just the proportions differ, otherwise these are the basic elements that the whole existence consists of.

> *The same object is seen in different ways by different* ·
> *minds . . . but a different mind will see the same*
> object in a different way.

For example, a woodcutter comes into the garden—he will not look at the flowers, he will not look at the greenery; he will be looking at the wood and the possibilities for the wood—which tree can become a beautiful table, which tree can become a door. For him, trees exist only as material for furniture. Potential furniture, that's what he will see. And if there comes a painter he will not think of furniture at all. Not even for a single moment will furniture enter into his consciousness. He will think of colors: the green, the red, the white, and thousands of colors all around. He will think of painting, of bringing these colors to canvas. If a poet comes he will not think of painting, he will think of something else. A philosopher comes and he will think still of something else. It depends on the mind. The object is always seen through the mind; the mind colors it.

Let me tell you a few anecdotes.

The tramp happened to call at the house of a temperance man. "I want to ask you a question," said the man to the tramp. "Do you ever take alcoholic drinks?" "Before I answer," said the tramp, "I want to know whether it is put as an inquiry or as an invitation."

It depends . . . the answer will depend on the question. The tramp is trying to be safe as to whether it is an invitation or an inquiry. His 'yes' and 'no' is going to be dependent on what it is. When you see a certain thing, you don't see the thing as such.

Immanuel Kant has said that a thing in itself cannot be known, and he is right in a way. He is right because whenever you know a thing, your mind, your prejudice, your greed, your concept, your culture, your religion, are all there looking at the thing. But Immanuel Kant is not absolutely true because there is a way to look at a thing without the mind. But he was not aware of meditation at all.

That's the difference between Western philosophy and Eastern philosophy. The Western philosophy goes on thinking through the mind, and the whole effort in the East is how to drop the mind and then see things, because then things appear in their own light, in their intrinsic qualities. Then you don't project anything.

He was the laziest man in the entire town. Unfortunately, he had a bad accident: he fell off his couch at home. A doctor examined him and said, "I'm afraid I have some rather bad news for you, sir. You will never be able to work again." "Thank you doctor," said the lazy one. "Now what is the bad news?"

For a lazy man it is not bad news that he will never be able to work again in his life. This is good news. It depends on your interpretation. And always remember, all interpretation is false because it falsifies reality.

The man lay on the psychiatrist's couch in a state of nervous tension. "I keep having this recurring, horrible nightmare," he told the psychiatrist. "In it I see my mother-in-law chasing me with a man-eating alligator on a leash. It is really frightening. I see the yellow eyes, the dry scaly skin, the yellow, decaying and razor-sharp teeth, and smell foetid heavy breath."

"It sounds pretty nasty," agreed the psychiatrist understandingly.

"That's nothing, doctor," continued the man. "Wait till I tell you about the alligator!"

Your mind is continuously projecting something. The reality functions as a screen and you go on working as a projector. A man who is learning how to be aware will learn how to drop his projections and look at facts as they are. Don't bring your mind in, otherwise you will never be able to know reality. You will remain closed in your own interpretations.

The same object is seen in different ways by different minds.
An object is not dependent on one mind.

But still, Patanjali is not saying the same things as Bishop Berkeley. Berkeley says that things are absolutely dependent on mind. He says that when you go out of your room everything in the room disappears. If there is nobody to see, how can things exist? And, in a way, it is difficult to disprove him because he says, "When you come back into the room again, things appear. When you go

out, they disappear because a mind is needed to interpret them."
Berkeley is saying that things are nothing but interpretations. So
when you go out, of course your interpretation goes with you and
there is no thing left in the room. It is very difficult to prove that he
is wrong, because if you come back into the room to prove, you
have come back, so things have appeared. But people have tried.
One man tried to find a few things which even Bishop Berkeley
would be forced to believe.

You are sitting in a train and the train is moving, and you are
not looking at the wheels, but still they are, because the train is
moving. Nobody may be looking at the wheels, but you cannot deny
that they are, otherwise you would not reach from one station to
another. And all the passengers are inside the train but nobody is
looking at the wheels, but wheels are. Of course, he was also
worried about things because if all things disappear, then how will
they come back again? Finally he decided that they exist in the
mind of God, so even when you are not there God is looking at your
furniture. That's why it remains; otherwise it would disappear.

Berkeley's philosophy is very logical in a way. He believes in the
mind, and he does not believe in matter. He says matter exists just
as things exist in your dreams. In your dream you see a palace; it
exists there, as real as anything you have ever seen. By the morning, when you open your eyes, it is gone. But when you dream it
again it is again there. He's a perfect *mayawadin*, a perfect believer
in illusion, that the world is illusory.

But Patanjali is very scientific. He says that the thing is not your
interpretation, though whatsoever you think about the thing is your
interpretation. The thing in itself exists. When nobody comes into
the garden—the carpenter, the woodcutter, the painter, the poet,
the philosopher; nobody comes into the garden—still flowers
flower, but without any interpretation. Nobody says they are beautiful, so they are not beautiful, they are not ugly. Nobody says they
are white or red, so they are not red or white, but still they are.

Things exist in themselves, but we can know things in themselves only when we have dropped our minds. Otherwise, our
minds go on playing tricks. We go on seeing things which we desire.
We see only that which we want to see. It happens every day here: I
talk to you; you listen to that which you want to listen to. You
choose that which helps you. Your own mind is strengthened by it.
If I say something which goes against you, there is every possibility
you will not listen to it. Or, even if you listen to it, you will
interpret it in such a way that it does not create any irritation in

your mind, that it is absorbed, that you make it a part of your mind. Whatsoever you hear has to be your interpretation, because you listen from the mind.

Patanjali says: right listening means listening without the mind, right seeing means seeing without the mind; you are simply aware.

An object is known or unknown depending on
whether the mind is colored by it or not.

Now, one thing more: when you look at an object, your mind colors the object and the object colors your mind. That's how things are known or unknown. When you look at a flower you say, "Beautiful." You have projected something on the flower. The flower is also projecting itself onto your mind: its color, its form. Your mind gets in tune with the form and the color of the flower; your mind gets colored by the flower. That's the only way to know a thing. If you are not colored by the flower, the flower may be there but you have not known it.

Have you watched?—you are in the market-place and somebody says, "Your house is on fire!" You start running, you pass by many people. Somebody says, "Hello, where are you going?" but you don't listen. On another day, at another time, you would have listened, but now your house is on fire. Your mind is totally directed towards your house. Now your attention is not here. You are not getting colored. You may pass a beautiful flower, but you will not say 'beautiful', you will not even recognize that the flower is there—impossible.

I have heard of one man, a very great philosopher; his name was Ishwar Chandra Vidyasagar. The Governor General was going to give him an award for his services, his learning, his scholarship, but he was a very poor man. He lived in Calcutta, a poor Bengali, and his clothes were not such that he should go wearing those clothes when the award was to be given to him. So the friends came and they said, "Don't be worried, we have ordered beautiful clothes for you." But he said, "I have never used anything more costly than these clothes. Just to take an award, should I change my whole way of life?" But the friends convinced him and he became ready. The same evening he was coming home from the market, just walking behind a Mohammedan who was walking with great dignity—very slow, with grace—a very beautiful man. And then a servant came running to that Mohammedan and said, "Sir, your house is on fire," but the Mohammedan continued the same way. The servant said,

"Have you heard me or not? Your house is on fire! Everything is burning!" The Mohammedan said, "I have heard you, but just because the house is on fire I cannot change my way of walking. And even if I run, I cannot save the house, so what is the point?"

Ishwar Chandra listened to this dialogue between the servant and the master. He could not believe his eyes, he could not believe his ears: "What is this man saying?" And then he remembered: "I am just changing my clothes and going in borrowed clothes just to receive an award?" He dropped the idea. The next day he appeared in his ordinary poor clothes. The Governor General asked, the friends asked; he related the story.

Now, this Mohammedan had a certain awareness, a certain awareness which cannot be clouded by anything, a certain wakefulness which is not easily disturbed. Ordinarily, everything colors you and you color everything. When this coloring stops, this reciprocal coloring stops, things start appearing in their true being. Then you come to see reality as it is. Then you come to know, 'This is It'. Then you come to know that which is.

These sutras are just indicators that unless a state of no-mind is achieved, ignorance cannot be destroyed. Awareness is against ignorance, knowledge is not against ignorance. So don't become parrots, and don't rely only on memorizing. Don't cram; try to see. Become more capable of seeing things as they are. The Vedas, the Upanishads, The Koran, the Bible, cannot help much. You can become great learned scholars, but you will remain, deep down, just fools. And when ignorance is decorated by knowledge then one clings to it. One does not want to destroy it. In fact, ego feels very happy.

You will have to choose. If you choose the ego, you will remain ignorant. If you want awareness, you will have to become aware of the tricks the ego goes on playing with you.

This morning, contemplate what you know and what you don't know, and don't be easily satisfied. Go as deep as possible into what you know and what you don't know. If you can decide that this you know and this you don't know, you have taken a great step. And that step is the most significant step a man can ever take because then the pilgrimage starts, the pilgrimage towards reality. If you go on believing that you know many things, and you don't know them, you are deceiving yourself and you will remain hypnotized by your knowledge. You will waste your whole life in drunkenness. Ordinarily, people live just like they are deeply asleep, walking in their sleep, doing things in their sleep, somnambulists.

Gurdjieff took Ouspensky and his thirty disciples to a very faraway place, and he told his thirty disciples to be absolutely silent for three months. He told them to be so silent that they should not communicate even through eyes or gestures. And thirty persons were to remain in a small bungalow as if there were not thirty people, but as if each one was living alone. After a few days a few people left, because it was too much, impossible. And Gurdjieff was a hard task-master. If he saw somebody smiling at somebody else, immediately he was expelled because he had communicated; the silence was broken. He said, "Live in this house as if you are alone. There are twenty-nine other people, but you are not concerned with them—just as if they are not." By the time the three months ended only three persons were left; twenty-seven had left. Ouspensky was one of those three persons. Those three persons became so silent that Gurdjieff took them outside the bungalow into the town, moved them in the market-place, and Ouspensky writes in his diary, "For the first time I could see that the whole of humanity is walking in sleep. People are talking in their sleep. Shopkeepers are selling things, customers are purchasing things, great crowds are going here and there, and I could see that moment that everybody is fast asleep; nobody is aware." He said, "We felt so uncomfortable in that mad place that we asked Gurdjieff to take us back to the bungalow. But he said, 'That bungalow was just an experiment to show you the reality of humanity, and you also have lived the same way. Because now you are silent you can see that people are just drunk, unconscious; not living really, just moving not knowing why, not knowing for what.' "

Watch yourself, meditate over it, and see whether you are living in sleep. If you are living in sleep, then come out of it.

Meditation is nothing but an effort to gather together the small consciousness that you have, to gather together, to crystallize it, to make all sorts of efforts to increase it more and more, and to decrease unconsciousness. By and by, consciousness becomes higher and higher: less and less dreamy; less and less thoughts come to you, and there are more and more gaps of silence. Through those gaps, windows will open to the divine. One day, when you have become really capable and you can say that, "I can exist for a few minutes without any thought or dream interfering with me," for the first time you will know. The purpose is fulfilled.

From deep sleep you have come to deep awareness. When deep sleep and deep awareness meet, the circle is complete.

That's what *samadhi* is. Patanjali calls it *kaivalya*—pure consciousness, alone; so pure, so alone that nothing else exists. Only in this aloneness does one become blissful. Only in this aloneness, one comes to know what truth is. Truth is your being. It is there but you are asleep.

Awake.

CHAPTER SIX
May 6, 1976

WITHOUT ANY CHOICE
OF YOUR OWN

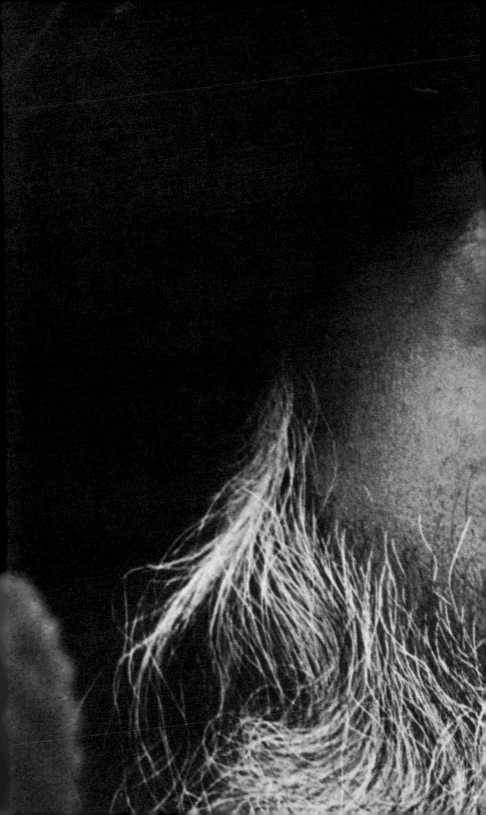

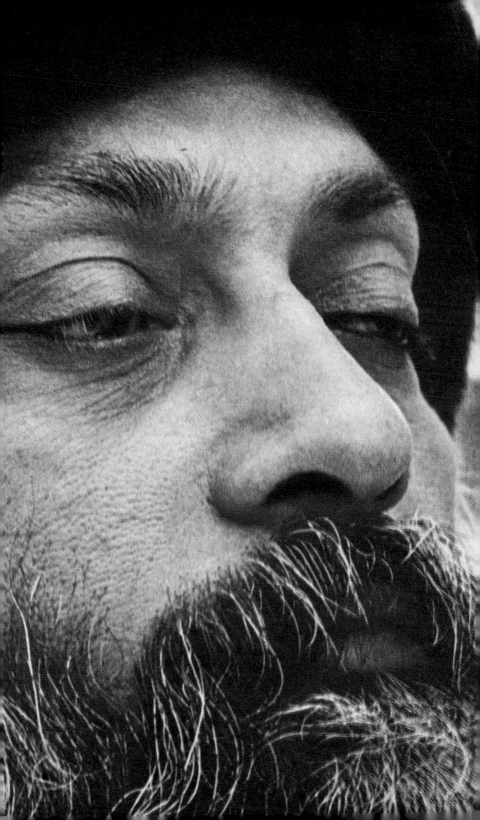

The first question:

Bhagwan, I was brought up in the teachings of Rudolph Steiner, but I could not yet break through my barriers towards him. Although I believe him to be right in the way he shows that for the West, the possibility to free ourselves from 'maya' is to learn to think in the right way. By doing this and by meditating, he says we are able to lose our egos and find our 'I'. The central figure for him is Christ, whom he differentiates from Jesus as a totally different being. Your way seems different to me. Can you please advise me? I am somehow torn between you and the way Steiner shows.

RUDOLPH STEINER WAS A GREAT MIND, but mind you, I say 'a great mind', and mind as such has nothing to do with religion. He was tremendously talented. In fact, it is very rare to find another mind to compare with Rudolph Steiner. He was so talented in so many directions and dimensions; it looks almost super-human: a great logical thinker, a great philosopher, a great architect, a great educator, and so on and so forth. And whatsoever he touched, he brought very novel ideas to that subject. Wherever he moved his eyes, he created new patterns of thought. He was a great man, a great mind, but mind as such, small or great, has nothing to do with religion.

Religion comes out of no-mind. Religion is not a talent, it is your nature. If you want to be a great painter, you have to be talented; if you want to be a great poet, you have to be talented; if you want to be a scientist, of course, you have to be talented; but if you want to be religious, no special talent is needed. Anybody, small or great, who is willing to drop his mind, enters into the dimension of the divine. And of course, great talented men find it very difficult to drop their minds; their investment is bigger. For an ordinary man who has no talent, it is very easy to drop the mind. Even then it seems so difficult. He has nothing to lose; still he goes on clinging. Of course, the difficulty is multiplied when you have a talented mind, when you are a genius. Then your whole ego is invested in your mind. You cannot drop it.

Rudolph Steiner founded a new movement called anthro-posophy, against theosophy. He was a theosophist in the beginning, then his ego started fighting other egos in the movement. He wanted to become the very head, the supreme-most of the theosophical movement in the world, the world head. That was not possible; there were many other egos. And the greatest problem was coming from J. Krishnamurti, who is not an ego at all. And of course, theosophists were thinking more and more towards Krishnamurti. He was becoming, by and by, the messiah. That created trouble in Rudolph Steiner's mind. He broke off from the movement. The whole German section of theosophy broke with him. He was really a very, very convincing orator, a convincing writer; he convinced people. He destroyed theosophy very badly, he divided it. And since then theosophy could never become whole and healthy.

Rudolph Steiner has an appeal for the Western mind, and that is the danger—because the Western mind is basically logic-oriented: reason, thinking, logos. He talks about it, and he says, "This is the way for the Western mind." No, Eastern or Western, mind is mind; and the way is no-mind. If you are Eastern, you will have to drop the Eastern mind. If you are Western, you will have to drop the Western mind. To move into meditation, mind, as such, has to be dropped. If you are a Christian you will have to drop a Christian mind. If you are a Hindu, you will have to drop the Hindu mind. Meditation is not concerned with Christian, Hindu, Eastern, West-ern, Indian or German, no.

What is mind? Mind is a conditioning given to you by the society. It is an over-imposition on the original mind, which we call no-mind. Just so that you don't get confused, all mind, as such, has to be dropped. The passage has to be completely empty for the divine to enter into you. Thinking is not meditation. Even right thinking is not meditation. Wrong or right, thinking has to be dropped. When there is no thought in you, no clouds of thinking in you, the ego disappears. And remember, when the ego disappears the 'I' is not found. The questioner says that Rudolf Steiner says, "When the ego disappears, the 'I' is found." No, when the ego disappears I is not found. Nothing is found. Yes, exactly; nothing . . . is found.

Just the other night I was telling a story of a great Zen master, To-san. He became empty, he became enlightened, he became a non-being; what Buddhists call *anatta*, no-mind. The rumor reached to the gods that somebody had again become enlightened.

And of course, when somebody becomes enlightened, gods want to
see his face—the beauty of it, the beauty of the original, the
virginity of it. Gods came down to the monastery To-san lived in.
They looked and looked, and they tried, and they would enter into
him from one side, and get out from another side, and nobody was
found inside To-san. They were very frustrated. They wanted to see
the face, the original face, and there was nobody. They tried many
devices, and then one very cunning god, clever, said, "Do one
thing": he ran into the kitchen of the monastery, brought handfuls
of rice and wheat. To-san was coming from his morning walk and
he threw it on his path.

In a Zen monastery, everything has to be respected absolutely;
even rice and wheat, stones, everything has to be respected. One
has to be continuously careful and aware. Not even a grain of rice
can you find in a Zen monastery lying here and there. You have to
be respectful. And remember, that respect has nothing to do with
Gandhian economics. It is not a question of economy, because
Gandhian economy is nothing but rationalized miserliness. It has
nothing to do with miserliness. It is a simple respect for everything,
absolute respect. This was disrespectful. This is the original idea of
the Upanishads where seers have said, *"Anambrahma"*—food is
God—because food gives you life, food is your energy. God comes
into your body through food, becomes your blood, your bones, so a
god should be treated as a god. When those gods threw rice and
wheat on the path where To-san came, he could not believe: "Who
has done this? Who has been so careless?" A thought arose in his
mind, and the story is that gods could see his face for a single
moment, because for a single moment the 'I' arose in a very subtle
way: "Who has done this? Something has gone wrong."

And whenever you decide what is wrong and what is right, you
are there, immediately. Between the right and the wrong exists the
ego. Between one thought and another thought exists the ego. Each
thought brings its own ego. For a moment, a cloud arose in To-san's
consciousness—"Who has done this?"—a tension. Each thought is a
tension. Even very ordinary, very innocent-looking thoughts are
tensions.

You see the garden is beautiful, and the sun is rising, and the
birds are singing, and an idea arises, "How beautiful!" Even that,
that is a tension. That's why if somebody is walking by your side,
you will immediately say to him, "Look, what a beautiful morning!" What are you doing? You are simply releasing the tension
that has come through the thought. Beautiful morning . . . a

thought has come; it has created a tension around it. Your being is no more non-tense. It has to be released, so you speak to the other. It is meaningless because he is also standing just where you are standing. He is also listening to the birds, he is also seeing the sun rise, he is also looking at the flowers, so what is the point of saying something like "this is beautiful"? Is he blind? But that is not the point. You are not communicating any message to him. The message is as clear to him as to you. In fact, you are relieving yourself of a tension. By saying it, the thought is dispersed into the atmosphere; you are relieved of the burden.

A thought arose in To-san's mind, a cloud gathered, and through that cloud the gods were able to see his face, just a glimpse. Again the cloud disappeared, again there was no longer any To-san.

Remember, this is what meditation is all about: to destroy you so utterly that even if gods come they cannot seek you, they cannot find you. You yourself have found when such a situation arises, that not even gods can find you. There is nobody inside to be found. That 'somebodiness' is a sort of tension. That's why people who think they are somebodies are more tense. People who think that they are nobodies are less tense. People who have completely forgotten that they are, are tensionless. So remember, when the ego is lost, the 'I' is not found. When the ego is lost nothing is found. That nothingness, that purity of nothingness is your being, your innermost core, your very nature, your Buddha-nature, your awareness—like a vast sky with no clouds gathered in it.

Now, listen to the question again.

"I was brought up in the teachings of Rudolph Steiner." Yes, they are teachings, and what I am doing here is not teaching you anything. Rather, on the contrary, I am taking all teachings away from you. I am not a teacher. I am not imparting knowledge to you. My whole effort is to destroy all that you think you know. My whole effort is to take all knowledge from you. I'm here to help you to unlearn.

"I was brought up in the teachings of Rudolph Steiner, but I could not yet break through my barriers towards him."

Nobody is able to break his barriers towards a person who is himself ego-oriented. It is difficult to break your barriers towards a person who is no more. Even then, it is so difficult to break your barriers because your ego resists. But when you are around a teacher who has his own ego-trip still alive, who *is* still, who is still trying to be somebody, who is still tense, it is impossible to drop down your ego.

"Although I believe him to be right in the way he shows that for the West, the possibility to free ourselves from *maya* is to learn to think in the right way."

No, the way for the East or for the West is: how to unlearn thinking, how not to think, and just be. And it is needed more for the West than for the East, because in the West the whole two millennia since Aristotle have been of conditioning you for thinking, thinking, thinking. Thinking has been the goal. The thinking mind has been the goal in the West: how to become more and more accurate, scientific· in your thinking. The whole scientific world arose out of this effort, because when you are working as a scientist you have to think. You have to work out in the objective world, and you have to find more accurate, exact, valid ways of thinking. And it has paid off too much. Science has been a great success, so of course people think that the same methodology will be helpful when you go inwards. That is the fallacy of Rudolph Steiner.

He thinks that in the same way as we have been able to penetrate into matter, the same method will help to go in. It cannot help, because to go in one has to move in just the opposite direction, diametrically opposite. If thinking helps to know matter, nothinking will help to know yourself. If logic helps to know matter, something like a Zen koan, something absurd, illogical, will help you to go in: faith, trust, love, maybe; but logic, never. Whatsoever has helped you to know the world better is going to be a barrier inside. And the same is true about the outer world also: whatsoever helps you to know yourself will not necessarily help you to know matter. That's why the East could not develop science.

The first glimpses of science had come to the East, but the East could not develop it. The East did not move in that direction. The basic rudimentary knowledge was developed in the East.

For example: mathematical symbols, figures from one to ten, were developed in India. That made mathematics possible. It was a great discovery, but there it stopped. The beginning happened, but the East could not go very far in that direction. Because of that, in all the languages of the world, the numerals, mathematical numerals, carry Sanskrit roots.

For example: two is Sanskrit *dwa*—it became twa, and then two. Three is Sanskrit *tri*—it became three. Six is Sanskrit *sasth*—it became six. Seven is Sanskrit *sapt*—it became seven. Eight is Sanskrit *ast*—it became eight. Nine is Sanskrit *nawa*—it became nine. The basic discovery is Indian, but then it stopped there.

In China they developed ammunition for the first time, almost five thousand years back, but they never made any bombs out of it. They made only fireworks. They enjoyed, they loved it, they played with it, but it was a toy. They never killed anybody through it. They never went too far into it.

The East has discovered many basic things, but has not gone deep into it. It cannot go, because the whole effort is to go within. Science is a Western effort; religion is an Eastern effort. In the West even religion tries to be scientific. That was what Rudolph Steiner was doing: trying to make the religious approach more and more scientific—because in the West, science is valuable. If you can prove that religion is also scientific, then religion also becomes valuable in a vicarious way, indirectly. So in the West, every religious person goes on trying to prove that science is not the only science, religion is also a science. In the East we have not bothered. It is just the other way round: if there was some scientific discovery, the people who had discovered it had to prove that it had some religious significance. Otherwise, it was meaningless.

"By doing this and by meditating, he says we are able to lose our ego and find our 'I'."

Rudolph Steiner does not know what meditation is, and what he calls meditation is concentration. He's completely confused: he calls concentration meditation. Concentration is not meditation. Concentration is again a very, very useful means for scientific thinking. It is to concentrate the mind, narrow the mind, focus the mind on a certain thing. But the mind remains, becomes more focused, becomes more integrated.

Meditation is not concentrating on anything. In fact, it is a relaxing, not narrowing. In concentration there is an object. In meditation there is no object at all. You are simply lost in an objectless consciousness, a diffusion of consciousness. Concentration is exclusive to something, and everything else is excluded from it. It includes only one thing; it excludes everything else.

For example: if you are listening to me you can listen in two ways: you can listen through concentration; then you are tense, and you are focused on what I am saying. Then the birds will be singing, but you will not listen to them. You will think that is a distraction.

Distraction arises out of your effort to concentrate. Distraction is a by-product of concentration. You can listen to me in a meditative way; then you are simply open, available—you listen to me, and you listen to the birds also, and the wind passes through the trees and creates a sound; you listen to that also—then you are simultaneously here. Then whatsoever is happening here, you are available to it without any mind of your own, without any choice of your own. You don't say, "I will listen to this and I will not listen to that." No, you listen to the whole existence. Then birds and me and the wind are not three separate things. They are not. They are happening simultaneously, together, all together, and you listen to the whole. Of course, then your understanding will be tremendously enriched because the birds are also saying the same thing in their way, and the wind is also carrying the same message in its way, and I am also saying the same thing in a linguistic way, so that you can understand it more. Otherwise, the message is the same. Mediums differ, but the message is the same, because God is the message.

When a cuckoo goes crazy, it is God going crazy. Don't exclude, don't exclude him; you will be excluding God. Don't exclude anything; be inclusive.

Concentration is a narrowing of consciousness; meditation is expansion: all doors are open, all windows are open, and you are not choosing. Then of course, when you don't choose you cannot be distracted. This is the beauty of meditation: a meditator cannot be distracted. And let that be the criterion: if you are distracted, know that you are doing concentration, not meditation. A dog starts barking—a meditator is not distracted. He absorbs that too, he enjoys that too. So he says, "Look . . . so God is barking in the dog. Perfectly good. Thank you for barking while I'm meditating. So you take care of me in so many ways," but no tension arises. He does not say, "This dog is antagonistic. He is trying to destroy my concentration. I am such a religious, serious man, and this foolish dog . . . what is he doing here?" Then enmity arises, anger arises. And you think this is meditation?—no, this is not of worth if you become angry at the dog, poor dog who is doing his own thing. He is not destroying your meditation or concentration or anything. He is not worried about your religion at all, nor about you. He may not even be aware of what nonsense you are doing. He's simply enjoying his way, his life. No, he is not your enemy.

Watch . . . if one person becomes religious in a house, the whole house becomes disturbed because that person is continuously on the verge of being distracted. He's praying; nobody should make any sound. He's meditating; children should remain silent, nobody should play. You are imposing unnecessary conditions on existence. And then if you are distracted and you feel disturbed, only you are responsible. Only you are to be blamed, nobody else.

What Rudolph Steiner calls meditation is nothing but concentration. And through concentration you can lose the ego and you will gain the 'I', and the 'I' will be nothing but a very, very subtle ego. You will become a pious egoist. Your ego will now be decorated in religious language, but it will be there.

"The central figure for him is Christ, whom he differentiates from Jesus as a totally different being."

Now, for a meditator there cannot be any central figure. There need not be. But for one who concentrates, something is needed to concentrate upon. Rudolph Steiner says Christ is the central figure. Why not Buddha? Why not Patanjali? Why not Mahavir? Why Christ? For Buddhists, Buddha is the central figure, not Christ. They all need some object to concentrate upon, something on which to focus their minds. For a religious man there is no central figure. If your own central ego has disappeared, or is disappearing, you need not have any other ego outside to support it. That Christ or Buddha is again an ego somewhere. You are creating a polarity of I-thou. You say, "Christ, thou art my master," but who will say this? An 'I' is needed to assert. Look, listen to Zen Buddhists. They say, "If you meet Buddha on the way, kill him immediately." If you meet Buddha on the way, *kill him immediately*, otherwise he will kill you. Don't allow him a single chance, otherwise he will possess you and he will become a central figure. Your mind will arise around him again. You will become a Buddhist mind. You will become a Christian mind. For a certain mind, a certain central object is needed.

And of course, he is more in favor of Christ than Jesus. That too has to be understood. That's how the pious ego arises. Jesus is just like us: a human being with a body, with ordinary life; very human. Now, for a very great egoist this won't do. He needs a very, very purified figure. Christ is nothing but Jesus purified. It is just like if you make curd out of your milk, then take cream out of it, and then you make *ghee* out of the cream. Then ghee is the purest part, the most essential. Now you cannot make anything out of ghee. Ghee is the last refinement, the white petrol. From kerosene, petrol; from petrol, white petrol. Now, no more; it is finished. Christ is just the purified Jesus. It is difficult for Rudolph Steiner to accept Jesus, and it is difficult for all egoists. They try to reject in many ways.

For example: Christians say that he was born out of a virgin. The basic problem is that Christians cannot accept that he was born just like we ordinary human beings. Then he will also look ordinary. He has to be special, and we have to be followers of a special

Master. Not like Buddha, born out of ordinary human love, ordinary human sexual copulation, no—Jesus is special. Special people need a special Master, out of a virgin. And he's the only begotten Son of God, the *only*. Because if there are other sons, then he is no longer special. He is the only Christ, the only one who has been crowned by God. All others, at the most, can be messengers, but cannot be of the same level and plane as Christ. Christians have done it in their own way, but I would like you to understand Jesus more than Christ—because Jesus will be more blissful to understand, peaceful to understand, and will be of great help on the path. Because you are in the situation of being a Jesus; Christ is just a dream.

First you have to pass through being a Jesus, and only then someday will Christ arise within you. Christ is just a state of being, just as Buddha is a state of being. Gautama became Buddha; Jesus became Christ. You can also become Christ, but right now Christ is too far. You can think about it and create philosophies and theologies about it, but that is not going to help. Right now it is better to understand Jesus, because that is where you are. That is from where the journey has to start. Love Jesus, because through loving Jesus you will love your humanity. Try to understand Jesus, and the paradox, and through that paradox you will be able to feel less guilty. Through understanding Jesus you will be able to love yourself more.

Now, Christians go on trying somehow to drop the paradox of Jesus through bringing the concept of Christ. For example: there are moments when Jesus is angry, and it is a problem; what to do? It is very difficult to avoid the fact because many times he is angry, and that goes against his very teaching. He continually talks about love, and is angry. And he talks about forgiving your enemies—not only that, but loving your enemies—but he himself lashes out his anger. In the temple of Jerusalem he took a whip, started beating the money changers, and threw them out of the temple single-handed. He must have been in a real fury, in a rage, almost mad. Now this . . . how to reconcile this? The way that Christians have found to reconcile—and Rudolph Steiner bases his own ideology on it—is to create a Christ, which is completely reconciled. Forget all about Jesus; bring a pure concept of Christ. You can say in that moment, "He was Jesus when he was angry." And when he said on the cross, "God my Father, forgive these people, because they don't know what they are doing," he was Christ. Now the paradox can be managed. When he was moving with women he was Jesus; when he told Magdalene not to touch him he was Christ. Two concepts help to figure things out—but you destroy the beauty of Jesus, because the whole beauty is in paradox.

There is no need to reconcile, because deep in Jesus' being they are reconciled. In fact, he could become angry because he loved so much. He loved so tremendously, that's why he could become angry. His anger was not part of hatred, it was part of his love. Have you not sometimes known anger out of love? Then where is the problem? You love your child: sometimes you spank the child, you beat the child, sometimes you are almost in a fury, but it is because of love. It is not because you hate. He loved so much— that's my understanding of Jesus—he loved so much that he forgot all about anger and he became angry. His love was so much. He was not just a dead saint, he was an alive person; and his love was not just philosophy, it was a reality. When love is a reality, sometimes love becomes anger also.

He was as human as you are. Yes, he was not finished there. He was more than human also, but first and basically he was human, human plus. Christians have been trying to prove that he was super-human and the humanity was just accidental, a necessary evil because he had to come into a body. That's why he was angry. Otherwise, he was just purity. That purity will be dead.

If purity is real and authentic, it is not afraid of impurity. If love is true it is not afraid of anger; if love is true it is not afraid of fighting. It shows that even fight will not destroy it; it will survive. There are saints who talk about loving humanity, but cannot love a single human being. It is very easy to love humanity. Always remember: if you cannot love, you love humanity. It is very easy, because you can never come across humanity, and humanity is not going to create any trouble. A single human being will create many troubles, many more. And you can feel very, very good that you love humanity. How can you love human beings?—you love humanity. You are vast, your love is great. But I will tell you: love a human being; that is the basic preparation for loving humanity. It is going to be difficult, and it is going to be a great crisis, a continuous crisis and challenge. If you can transcend it, and you don't destroy love because of the difficulties but you go on strengthening your love so that it can face all difficulties—possible, impossible—you will become integrated. Christ loved human beings, and loved so much, and his love was so great that it transcended human beings and became the love for humanity. Then it transcended humanity and became love for existence. That is love for God.

"Your way seems different to me."

Not only different; it is diametrically opposite. In the first place,
it is not a way at all. It is not a path, or if you love the word then
call it a pathless path, a gateless gate. But it is not a path, because
a path or way is needed if your reality is far away from you. Then it
has to be joined by a path. But my whole insistence is that your
reality is available to you right now. It is just within you. A path is
not needed to reach to it. In fact, if you drop all paths, you will
suddenly find yourself standing in it. The more you follow paths,
the farther away you go from yourself. Paths misguide, mislead,
because you are already that which you are seeking. So paths are
not needed, but if you are trained to think in those terms, then I
will say that my way is diametrically opposite. Steiner says right-
thinking; and I say, right or wrong, all thinking is wrong. Thinking
as such is wrong; no-thinking is right.

"Can you please advise me? because I am somehow torn between
you and the way Steiner shows."

No, you will have to remain in that state of tension for a few
days. I will not advise and I will not help. Because if I advise and I
help you, you can come and lean towards me; that may be imma-
ture. You will have to have a good fight with Steiner before you can
come to me, and he will certainly give you a good fight. He is not
going to leave you so easily. And I'm not going to give you any help,
so that you come on your own. Only then do you come, when you
come on your own. When a fruit is ripe it falls on its own accord.
No, I will not throw even a small stone at it, because the fruit may
not be ripe and the stone may bring it down . . . and that will be a
calamity. You would remain in your torn state of mind.

You will have to decide, because nobody can remain in a torn
state of mind for long. There is a point where one has to decide.
And it will not be just towards Rudolph Steiner if I help you. He's
dead; he cannot fight with me. It is easier for me to pull you
towards me than it will be for him. So to also be just to him it is
better that I leave it to you. You just go on fighting. Either you will
drop me . . . that will also be a gain, because then you will follow
Rudolph Steiner more totally.

But I don't think that is possible now . . . the poison has entered
you. Now it is only a question of time.

✝

The second question:

When I am with the plants, rivers, mountains, animals, birds, sky, I feel okay. But when I come among the people I feel as if I have come into the madhouse. Why is this division?

When you are with trees, the sky, the river, the rocks, the flowers, and you feel okay, it has nothing to do with you. It has something to do with the trees and the river and the rocks. That okay-ness comes from their silence. When you come close to human beings you start feeling mad, in a madhouse, because human beings are mirrors; they reflect you. You must be mad. That's why you feel when you are with people that you are in a madhouse. I have never felt that way. Even with mad people like you I have never felt that way.

This is one of the basic problems every religious seeker comes to confront.

When you are alone things seem to be settled, because there is nobody to disturb. Nobody gives a chance for you to be disturbed. Everything is silent, so you also feel a certain silence, but this silence is natural. It is nothing spiritual. It belongs to nature. If you go to the Himalayas, to the cool, hushed silence of the Himalayan peaks, you will feel silent. But the credit goes to the Himalayas, not to you. When you come back, you will come back the same man who had gone. You will not be able to carry the Himalayas with you. So many have gone there and remained there forever, thinking that now, if they went back to the world they would lose something that they had attained. They had not attained anything. Because once you attain it, it cannot be lost; and the world is the test. So if you feel good while there are no human beings, it simply shows that amidst human beings your inner madness starts functioning. So don't become an escapist, and don't blame the society, the people, the crowd. Don't say that it is a madhouse. Rather, start thinking that you must be carrying mad tendencies within you which become manifest when you come into relationship with people.

Two psychiatrists pass each other on the street. One says, "Hello." The other says, "Now, I wonder what he means by that?"

Just a small thing like somebody saying hello, and a problem arises . . . "Now, I wonder what he means by that?"

The patient told his doctor that he kept seeing spots in front of his eyes. The doctor told him to stop going out with freckled women. Then he told him to stick his tongue out as he left. "Why?" asked the patient. "Because I hate my nurse."

Patients and doctors are all in the same boat.

Of course, when you come amongst people, you come amongst people like you. Suddenly, something in you starts responding. They are mad; you are mad—the moment you come close, a subtle dialogue of energy starts happening. Your madness brings their madness out; their madness brings your madness out. If you live alone, you are happy.

Mulla Nasrudin was saying to me, "I and my wife lived for twenty-five years tremendously happily." I asked, "Then what happened?" He said, "Then we met; since then, no happiness."

Even two happy persons meet and immediately unhappiness arises. You are carrying subtle seeds of unhappiness in you. The right opportunity, and they sprout. And of course, for a human being to sprout in all his potentialities, a human environment is needed. Trees don't make your environment. You can go to a tree and sit silently and do whatsoever you like; you remain unrelated. There exists no dialogue, no language between you and the tree. The tree goes on brooding in his own being, and you go on brooding in your own being. No bridge exists. A river is a river; no bridge exists between you and the river. When you come near a human being, suddenly you see you are bridged, and that bridge starts immediately transferring things from this side to that, from that side to this.

But basically it is you, so don't blame the society, don't blame people. They simply reveal you. And if you are a little understanding, you will thank them for doing a great thing for you. They reveal you; they show you who you are, where you are, what you are. If you are mad, they show your madness. If you are a Buddha, they show your Buddha-hood. Alone, you don't have any reference. Alone, you don't have any contrast. Alone, you cannot know who you are.

I will tell you one very beautiful story, a sad story.

The situation was not unusual. The boss of a large and successful firm employed a beautiful secretary. The boss, in his early forties, was a bachelor. He had a large car, a luxury flat, and was never short of feminine company. But he met his match in his beautiful secretary. She politely refused his invitations to lunch or dinner, and his offers of expensive presents and salary increases were refused with equal grace and charm. In the early weeks of her employment, he was of the opinion that she was just playing hard-to-get. During the months that followed, he changed his toothpaste, his soap, his after-shave, but all to no avail. Finally, he resigned himself to accept the fact that she was beautiful and highly competent, but that his chances of developing any kind of personal relationship with her were nil. It therefore came as something of a shock when he walked into his office one morning and found his secretary arranging flowers on his desk, and even more of a shock when she looked at him demurely and said, "A happy birthday, sir." He mumbled his thanks and went through the rest of the day in a complete daze. As the time approached five o'clock, the secretary came into the office and confessed that she had ascertained his birthday from the staff files. "I hope you don't mind," she added. He answered that he didn't mind it at all, and she looked relieved. "In that case, sir," she went on, "I wonder if you would care to come round to my flat this evening, at about nine o'clock. I have got a little surprise for you that I think you will find very pleasant." He mentally congratulated himself on the fact that the girl had finally had to admit that she was attracted to him, and tried to appear casual as the arrangements were finalized. Promptly at nine o'clock, a bottle of champagne in his hand, he presented himself at the flat. She was a vision of loveliness, and he hoped that she could not hear his heart pounding as she poured him a large scotch and urged him to make himself comfortable. "Loosen some of your clothes if you are too warm," she said. "I'm just going into the bedroom to get ready. Please come too when I call you." This was too good to be true. "I must be as desirable to her as she is to me," he thought smugly. "You can come in now," she called eventually, "but be careful you don't fall. All the lights are off in here." Our hero could take a hint. Quickly slipping out of his clothes, he entered the darkened room and closed the door behind him. As he did so the room became flooded with light and he saw that the whole of the office staff stood in the center of the room singing, "Happy birthday to you. . . ."

People reveal only that which you are hiding within you. If you feel that you are in a madhouse, you must be mad. Try to be in company more with men; try to be in company more with women; try to be with people more. Try more relationships. If you cannot be happy with a human being, it is impossible for you to be happy with a tree or with a river—impossible. If you cannot understand a human being who is so close to you, so similar to you, how can you hope that you will be able to understand a tree, a river, a mountain, who are so far away? Millions of years separate you from a mountain. You may have been a mountain somewhere millions of lives before, but you have completely forgotten the language. And the mountain cannot understand your language. The mountain has yet to become human: a long evolution is needed. A vast abyss exists between you and the mountain. If you cannot bridge yourself with human beings who are so close, so close, then it is impossible for you to bridge with anything else.

First, bridge yourself with human beings. By and by, the more you become capable of understanding human beings, the more you become capable of an inner dialogue, harmony, rhythm. Then you can move, by and by. Then move to animals; that is a second step. Then move to birds, then move to trees, then move to rocks, and only then can you move to pure existence, because that is the source. And we have been away from that source so long and so far away that we have completely forgotten that we ever belonged to it, or that it ever belonged to us.

The third question:

Beloved Bhagwan, I hear you, your loving compassion for me as a woman, behind your words, which sometimes jar me. And I also feel that my very woman-ness is the main barrier to my ever experiencing the bliss of enlightenment, because all of the enlightened beings you ever talk about are men, and because your own experiences are as a male. Please share with me what you can about how enlightenment is for me as a woman.

First thing: womanliness is never a barrier to understanding. In fact, you cannot find a better opportunity to understand me. It is difficult for a man to understand because a man has an aggressive mind. A man can easily become a scientist, but it is very difficult for him to become a religious person because religion needs receptivity, a passive state of consciousness where you don't aggress, just invite. The feminine mind is exactly the right mind to understand, to be a disciple. Even a male mind has to become feminine. So don't take it as a barrier; it is not.

The second thing: it is really a great problem because we don't understand it. Problems are there only because we don't understand them. Again and again it is asked of me, that I am always talking about men who become enlightened but never about women. Many women have become enlightened, as many as men. Nature keeps a certain balance. Watch . . . in the world, the number of men and women is almost always the same. It should not be so, but nature keeps balance. To one person there may be born only boys, ten boys; to another person only one boy may be born; to another, one girl—but on the whole, the world always keeps balance. There are as many men as there are women. Not only that, but because a woman is stronger than a man—stronger in the sense of her resistance, stability, capacity to adjust, flexibility—to a hundred girls, one hundred and fifteen boys are born. But by the time those girls become marriageable, fifteen boys have disappeared. Boys die more than girls; nature keeps that too. A hundred girls and one hundred and fifteen boys are born, then fifteen boys disappear by the time they become marriageable. The balance is kept completely. Not only that, but in wartime more men die.

The First World War created a problem for psychologists, biologists. They could not believe what had happened. In a war, more men die, but immediately after the war, more men are born and less girls are born. Again the balance is kept. That happened in the First World War. The reason was not clear at all. It was simply a mystery. It happened again in the Second World War. After a war the number of boys becomes greater. More boys are born to replace the dead men, and less girls are born because already there are more girls alive. When the World War is over and the balance is again regained, the number comes back to the same old pattern: one hundred girls to one hundred and fifteen boys—because fifteen boys will die.

Boys are less strong than girls. Men live five years less than women. That's why, in the world, you will always find more old women than old men, more widows than widowers. If the average age for a woman is eighty, then the average for men is seventy-five. It is five years more. But why, why do women live five years more? That too seems to be a great inner balance somewhere. A woman is capable of accepting more than a man. If a man dies first, the woman will cry, weep, suffer, but will be able to accept the fact. She will regain balance. But if a woman dies the man cannot regain balance. The only way he knows to regain balance is to marry again, find another woman again; he cannot live alone. He's more helpless than a woman.

Ordinarily, all over the world the marriage age is somehow

unnatural. Everywhere man has imposed a pattern which is un-natural, anti-nature. If the girl is twenty years of age, then we think that the age of the boy who is going to marry her should be twenty-five, twenty-six. It should be just the reverse, because later on girls are going to live five more years. So the age limit for the girls should be twenty-five if it is twenty for the boys. Every man should marry a woman who is at least five years older than him. Then the balance will be perfect. Then they will die almost within six months of one another, and there will be less suffering in the world.

But why has it not happened?—because marriage is not a natural thing. Otherwise, nature would have managed it that way. It is a man-made institution. And man feels a little weak if he is going to marry a woman who is older, more experienced, more knowledgeable than him. He wants to keep his male chauvinist ego: he's greater in every way. No man wants to marry a woman who is taller than him. Nonsense. What is the point? Why not marry a woman who is taller than you? But the male ego feels hurt moving with a taller woman. Maybe this is the cause of why women don't grow so tall—the feminine body has learned it. They have learned the trick, that they have to be a little shorter, otherwise they will not be able to find a man. It is a survival of the fittest. They fit only when they are not too tall. A very tall woman . . . just think of a woman seven feet tall; she will not find a husband. She will die without a husband. And she will not give birth to children, so she will disappear. A woman who is five feet five will find a man easily. She will survive: she will have a husband, she will have children. Of course, taller women will disappear, by and by, because they will not have any survival value. That's how, by and by, ugly women disappear from the world—because they cannot survive. The world helps those who can survive, and those who cannot survive disappear. Man has become taller, stronger, but in every way he wants to keep himself a little higher than the woman. He should always be at the top of everything.

Even in the West, people had not heard of any woman making love on top of the man before coming to the East and coming across Vatsayana's sutras on sexology. The West had not known it. And in the East, you may be surprised to know that the man making love on top of a woman is called the missionary posture, because the East for the first time came to know about it through Christian missionaries. It is a missionary posture. Man has to be on top in every way, even while making love. He has to have a taller height,

more age, more education. If you are going to marry a woman who
is a Ph.D., you will feel a little uneasy if you are not a Ph.D. You
must be at least a D.Lit.; only then can you marry a Ph.D. woman.
Otherwise, naturally, a woman has to be five years older than the
man. And this seems to be a perfect arrangement because the
woman needs to be more experienced. She is going to become the
mother: not only the mother of her children, but the mother of her
husband also. And a man remains childish. Whatsoever the age,
he hankers to be a child again. He remains a little juvenile.

Now the same has happened with enlightenment also—nature
keeps an exact balance. But we don't hear about many enlightened
women—that's true—because the society belongs to men. They
don't record much about women. They record much about Buddha;
they don't record much about Sahajo. They record much about
Mohammed; they don't record much about Rabia. They record in
such a way that men seem to be very prominent. It has happened in
India: one Jain Teerthankara, one Jain Master, an enlightened man,
was not a man; she was a woman. Her name was Mallibai, but a
great following of Jains has changed her name. They call her
Mallinath, not Mallibai. *Bai* shows that she was a woman; *nath*
shows that she was a man.

There are two sects of Jains, *Swetambaras* and *Digambaras*.
Digambaras say that she was not a woman: Mallinath. They have
even changed her name. It seems to be against the male ego that a
woman could become a Teerthankara, a great Master: enlightened,
a founder of a religion, a founder of a ford towards the divine? No,
it is not possible. They have changed the name.

History is recorded by men, and women are not interested in
recording things. They are more interested in experiencing and
living them: that is one thing. The second thing is that a woman
finds it very easy to become a disciple, *very* easy to become a
disciple, because she is receptive. For a man, it is difficult to
become a disciple because he has to surrender, and that is the
trouble. He can fight but he cannot surrender. So when it comes to
disciplehood, women are perfect. But just the opposite happens
when you have to become a Master.

A male can easily become a Master. A woman finds it very
difficult to become a Master, because to become a Master you have
to be really aggressive. You have to go out and destroy others'
structures. You have to be almost violent; you have to kill your
disciples. You have to brainwash them. So a woman finds it
difficult to become a Master; a man finds it difficult to become a

disciple. But then again there is a balance: women find it easier to become disciples, and by becoming disciples they become enlightened, but they never become Masters. A man finds it difficult to become a disciple, but once he becomes a disciple, is enlightened, it is very easy for him to become a Master, very easy for him, easier. That's why you never hear ... but don't be worried about that.

Your own experiences are as a female. Remember, the experience of the ultimate has nothing to do with male and female. The experience of the ultimate is beyond the duality. So when you become enlightened, in that moment you are no more man or woman. In that moment you transcend all duality. You have become a complete circle; no division exists. So when I am talking to you, I am not talking about enlightenment as a man. Nobody can talk about enlightenment as a man because enlightenment is neither male nor female. In India, the ultimate reality is neither male nor female, it is neutral.

You will be in a difficulty: God is male in the Western mind. For God you use 'He'—except for the Lib. Movement women, who have started to use 'She'. Otherwise, nobody uses 'She' for God; you use 'He'. And I also think that 'She' will be better. 'He' has been used enough; now 'She' will be better. 'She' includes 'He'—after 's' there is 'he'—but 'he' does not include 's'. It is better, it makes God a little bigger. 'She' is bigger than 'He'; nothing is wrong in it.

But in the Western mind, God is 'He'. In Western languages there are only two genders, male and female. In Indian languages, particularly in Sanskrit, we have three genders: male, female, and the neutral. God is neutral. He is neither He nor She; He is It, That—the personality has disappeared. It is impersonal, just energy. So don't be worried about this either.

"Please share with me what you can about how enlightenment is for me as a woman."

Stop thinking about yourself as a woman, otherwise you will cling to the feminine mind. *All* minds have to be dropped. In deep meditation you are neither. In deep love also, you are neither. Have you watched it?

If you have made love to a woman or to a man, and the love was really total and orgasmic, you forget who you are. It is mind-blowing. You simply don't know who you are. In a certain moment of deep orgasmic bliss, oneness happens. That is the whole effort of Tantra: to transform sex into an experience of oneness—because that will be your first experience of oneness, and enlightenment is the last experience of oneness. Making love, you disappear—the man becomes like woman, the woman becomes like man, and many times they change roles. And there comes a moment, if you are both in a total let-go, when a circle of energy arises which is neither. Let that be your first experience. Love is the basic experience of enlightenment, a first glimpse. Then one day, when you and the whole meet in a deep orgasm, that is *samadhi*, ecstasy. Then you are no more male or female. So from the very beginning start dropping the division.

In the Western consciousness the division has become very, very solid, because man has oppressed woman so much that the woman has to resist. And she can resist only if she becomes more and more conscious of being a woman. When you from the West come to me, it is going to be hard for you, but you have to understand and drop the man/woman division. Just be beings. And my whole effort here is to make you your original being, which is neither.

The last question:

I feel as if I had no choice in coming to you. Do we really ever choose things that happen in our lives?

Ordinarily, no. Ordinarily you move like a robot, a mechanical thing, accidental. Unless you become perfectly aware you cannot choose. And there comes the paradox: you can become aware only if you become choiceless; and if you become aware, you become capable of choice. You can choose—because when you are aware, you can decide what to do and what not to do. Ordinarily, you live almost in a state of drunkenness. A somnambulist, that's what you are.

Let me tell you a few anecdotes.

A minister was bemoaning to a friend that he had had his bicycle stolen.

And the friend said, "Well, next Sunday, why don't you use the Ten Commandments as your text and recite them to the congregation? When you reach the one that says 'Thou shalt not steal', have a look at the congregation, and if the thief is present he will probably give himself away by the expression on his face."

The following week the same friend saw the minister cycling through the village and stopped him. "I see that you got your bike back. My idea worked then?"

"Well, not exactly," said the minister. "I started on the Ten
Commandments, but when I got to the one that says 'Thou shalt
not commit adultery', I remembered where I had left my bike."
Another anecdote.

An eminent businessman went to the doctor. "Doctor," he said,
"I wish to consult you about my son. I believe he has got measles."

"There is a great deal of it about at the moment," said the
doctor. "No family seems to be safe from it."

"But doctor," he went on, "the boy said he got it from kissing the
maid, and to tell the truth, I'm afraid I'm also in danger from the
same disease. And what is worse, every night I kiss my wife, so she
may be in danger."

"Good heavens!" said the doctor. "Excuse me, I must go and get
my throat examined at once!"

Get it?

Everybody is moving in an unconscious circle, and people are
exchanging their illnesses, diseases, their unconscious, sharing only
their unconsciousness with each other.

Ordinarily you live as if you are asleep. You cannot decide while
you are asleep. How can you decide?

A man came to Buddha and said, "I would like to serve humanity." He must have been a great philanthropist. Buddha looked at
him, and it is said that tears came to Buddha's eyes. It was strange.
Buddha crying?—for what? The man also felt very uncomfortable.
He said, "Why are you crying? Have I said anything wrong?"
Buddha said, "No, not anything wrong. But how can you serve
humanity?—you are not yet. I see you fast asleep; I can hear your
snoring. That's why I am crying. And you want to serve humanity?
The first thing is to become aware, alert. The first thing is, to be."

The beautiful but dumb secretary got away with murder as far
as her boss was concerned. But one morning he really lost his
temper with her. "You are late again!" he thundered. "Why don't
you use the alarm clock that I bought for you?"

"But I do use it," she pouted prettily. "Every night."

"Well," said the boss, "why don't you get up when it goes off?"

"But it always goes off when I'm asleep!"

This is what's happening. You are asleep, and when you are
asleep even an alarm clock cannot help much. Have you sometimes
observed the fact that if you are asleep and the alarm clock goes off,
you start dreaming some dream: a dream that you are in a temple
and the temple bells are ringing? To avoid the fact that the alarm
clock is ringing, you create a dream around it. Then, of course, you

continue asleep; now there is no alarm clock. That's what is happening continuously to you. You go on listening to me, but I know that you will create a dream around it. If you listen to me you are bound to awake, but the problem is, will you listen to me? Will you create some dream around what I say?

And you create dreams. You can create a dream about enlightenment. You can start dreaming about enlightenment; you have missed me. And people go on missing. The message has to be interpreted by you; that's the trouble.

I have heard: The owner of a large company bought a sign which said "Do it now", and hung it up in the office hoping it would inspire his staff with promptness. A few days later a friend asked him if the notice had had any effect. "Well, not in the way I had hoped," admitted the boss. "The cashier absconded with $10,000—Do it now—the head bookkeeper eloped with my private secretary—Do it now—three clerks asked for a raise, a typist threw her typewriter out of the window—Do it now—and the office boy has ... just ... aah ... poisoned my coffee ... aaah!"

You listen through your sleepiness; you will interpret it in your own way. So if you really want to listen to me, don't interpret.

Just the other night, a new young man became a sannyasin. I told him, "Be here for a few days." He said, "But I am going, just within two or three days." I said, "But that is not right. Much has to be done, and you have just come. You have not had even any contact with me yet. So at least be here for the camp and a few days more." He said, "I will think it over." Then I told him, "Then there is no need to think; you go. Because whatsoever you will think is going to be wrong. And the whole point of sannyas is that you start listening to me without thinking about it. The whole point is that I say something to you, and it becomes more important than your own mind. That is the whole meaning of sannyas. Now if there is a conflict between what I say and your mind, you will drop the mind and you will listen to me. That's the risk. If you continuously go on using your mind to decide even whether what I say has to be done or not, then you remain yourself. You don't come out. You don't bring your hand close to me so that I can hold it."

Ordinarily, everything is happening to you; you have not done anything.

"I feel as if I had no choice in coming to you."

That's perfectly true. You must have drifted in some way. A friend was coming to me and he told you, or you just went to a bookstall and you found a book of mine.

One sannyasin came and I asked him, "How did you come to see me? How in the first place did you become interested?" He said, "I was sitting in Goa, on the beach, and just in the sand I found a *Sannyas* magazine that somebody must have left. So, nothing to do, I started reading it. That's how I have come here." Accidental. . . .

You have come to me accidentally, but now there is an opportunity to be alertly with me, to be with me with full awareness. It is good that accidentally you have come to me, but don't remain here accidentally. Now drop that accidental-ness. Now, take charge of your awareness. Otherwise, somebody will take you again, accidentally, somewhere else. Again you will drift away from me—because one who has come drifting cannot be relied upon. He will drift; something else will happen. Somebody is going to Nepal and the idea occurs to you, "Why not go to Nepal?" and you go to Nepal. And there you meet a girlfriend who is against sannyas, so what to do? You have to drop your sannyas.

Now that you are here, use this opportunity. People also use opportunities only in a very unconscious way. Use it consciously.

The magistrate said, "What induced you to strike your wife?" The husband said, "Well, your Honour, she had her back to me, the frying pan was handy, the back door was open, and I was slightly drunk, so I thought I would take a chance."

People use their opportunities also in an unconscious way. Use this opportunity in a conscious way, because this opportunity is such that it can be used *only* consciously.

CHAPTER SEVEN
May 7, 1976

THE WITNESS IS
SELF-ILLUMINATING

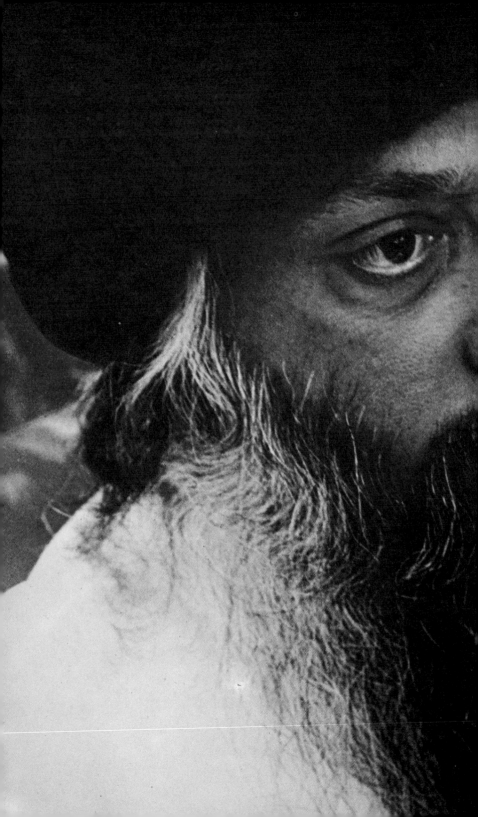

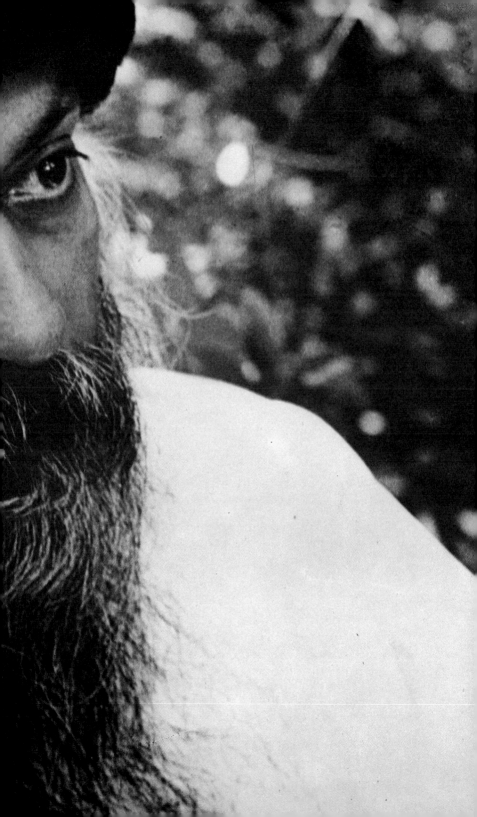

18

The modifications of the mind are always known by its lord, due to the constancy of the Purusa, pure consciousness.

सदा ज्ञाताश्चित्तवृत्तयस्तत्प्रभोः पुरुषस्यापरिणामित्वात् ॥ १८ ॥

19

The mind is not self-illuminating, because it is itself perceptible.

न तत्स्वाभासं दृश्यत्वात् ॥ १९ ॥

20

It is impossible for the mind to know itself and any other object at the same time.

एकसमये चोभयानवधारणम् ॥ २० ॥

21

If it were assumed that a second mind illuminates the first, cognition of cognition would also have to be assumed, and a confusion of memories.

चित्तान्तरदृश्ये बुद्धिबुद्धेरतिप्रसङ्गः स्मृतिसंकरश्च ॥ २१ ॥

22

Knowledge of its own nature through self-cognition is obtained when consciousness assumes that form in which it does not pass from place to place.

चितेरप्रतिसंक्रमायास्तदाकारापत्तौ स्वबुद्धिसंवेदनम् ॥ २२ ॥

23

When the mind is colored by the knower and the known, it is all-apprehending.

द्रष्टृदृश्योपरक्तं चित्तं सर्वार्थम् ॥ २३ ॥

24

Though variegated by innumerable desires, the mind acts for another, for it acts in association.

तदसंख्येयवासनाभिश्चित्रमपि परार्थं संहत्यकारित्वात् ॥ २४ ॥

The first sutra:

*The modifications of the mind are always known by
its lord, due to the constancy of the Purusa, pure
consciousness.*

PATANJALI TAKES THE WHOLE COMPLEXITY OF THE
HUMAN BEING INTO ACCOUNT; that has to be understood. Never before and never after has such a comprehen-
sive system ever been evolved. Man is not a simple being.
Man is a very complex organism. A rock is simple because the rock
has only one layer, the layer of the body. It is what Patanjali calls
anamayakos: the most gross, only one layer. You go into the rock;
you will find layers of rock but nothing else. Look at a tree and you
will also find something else other than the body. The tree is not
just the body. Something of the subtle has happened to it. It is not
so dead as rock; it is more alive—a subtle body has come into
existence. If you treat a tree like a rock, you mistreat it. Then you
have not taken into account the subtle evolution that has happened
between the rock and the tree. The tree is highly evolved. It is more
complex. Then, take an animal—still more complex. Another layer
of subtle body has evolved.

Man has five bodies, five seeds, so if you really want to understand man and his mind—and there is no way of going beyond if
you don't understand the whole complexity—then we have to be
very patient and careful. If you miss one step, you will not be able
to reach to your innermost core of being. The body that you can see
in the mirror is the outermost shell of your being. Many have
mistaken it, as if this is all.

In psychology, there is a movement called behaviorism, which
thinks that man is nothing but the body. Always beware of people
who talk of 'nothing buts'. Man is always more than any 'nothing
but' can imply. Behaviorists: Pavlov, B. F. Skinner and company,
think that man is the body—not that you have a body, not that you
are in the body, but simply that you are the body. Then man is
reduced to the lowest denominator. And of course, they can prove
it. They can prove it because that is the most gross part of man and
is easily available to scientific experimentation. The subtle layers of
man's being are not so easily available. Or, to say it in other words:

scientific instrumentation is not yet so sophisticated. It cannot touch the subtler layers of man.

Freud, Adler, go a little deeper into man. Then man is not just the body. They touch something of the second body, what Patanjali calls *pranamayakos:* the vital body, the energy body. But only a very fragmentary part is touched by Freud and Adler; one part by Freud and another part by Adler.

Freud reduces man to just sexuality. That is also there in man, but that is not the whole story. Adler reduces man to just ambition, will to power. That too is there in man. Man is very big, very complex. Man is an orchestra; many instruments are involved in it.

But this has always happened. This is a calamity, but this has always happened: when once somebody finds something, he tries to make a total philosophy out of his finding. That's a great temptation. Freud stumbled upon sex, and that too, not the whole of sex. He stumbled only upon the repressed sexuality. He came across repressed people. Christian repression has made many blocks in man where energy has become coiled up within itself, has become stagnant, is no longer flowing. He came against those rock-like blocks in the stream of human energy, and he thought—and the ego always thinks that way—that he had found the ultimate truth. Adler, working in a different way, stumbled upon another block of man: the will to power. And then he made a whole philosophy out of it.

Man has been taken in fragments. Yoga is the only philosophy in existence which takes the whole of man into account. Jung went still a little further, deeper. One fragment of the third body of man, *manomayakos*—he caught hold of it and he created a whole philosophy out of it. To comprehend the whole body—even that has not been possible because the body itself is very complex: millions of cells in a great harmony, functioning in a miraculous way. When you were born in your mother's womb, you were just a small cell. Out of that one cell, another cell arises. The cell grows and divides in two, then the two cells grow and divide into four. Out of one division—and division goes on—you have millions of cells. And they all function in a deep cooperation, as if somebody is holding them. It is not a chaos; you are a cosmos.

And then, some cells become your eyes, some cells become your ears, some cells become your genital organs, some cells become your skin, some cells your bones, some cells your brain, some cells your nails and your hair; and they all are coming out of one cell. They are all alike. They have no qualitative difference, but they function so differently. The eye can see; the ear cannot see. The ear can hear, but cannot smell. So those cells not only function in harmony, but they become experts. They gain to a certain special-ization. A few cells turn into the eyes. What has happened? What type of training is going on? Why do certain cells become eyes, and certain other cells become ears, and still certain others become your nose, and they are all alike? There must be a great training inside—some unknown power training them for a specific purpose.

And remember, when those cells are getting ready to see, they have not yet seen anything. When the child is in the womb, he remains completely blind. He has not seen any light; the eyes are closed. A miracle: no training to see and the eyes are ready, no possibility to see and the eyes are ready. The child does not breathe with his own lungs, he has not known what breathing is, but the lungs are ready. They are ready before the child is going to enter into the world and breathe. The eyes are ready before the child is going to enter into the world and see. Everything is ready. When the child is born he is a perfect human being of tremendous complexity, specialization, subtlety. And there has been no train-ing, no rehearsal. The child has never taken a single breath, but immediately out of the mother's womb, he cries and takes his first breath. The mechanism is ready before any training has been given: some tremendous power, some power which comprehends all the possibilities of the future, some power which is preparing the child to be able to face all possibilities of life for the future, is working deep within.

Even the body is not completely understood, not yet. Our whole understanding is fragmentary. The science of man does not exist yet. Patanjali's yoga is the closest effort ever made. He divides the body into five layers, or into five bodies. You don't have one body, you have five bodies; and behind the five bodies, your being. The same as has happened in psychology has happened in medicine. Allopathy believes only in the physical body, the gross body. It is parallel to behaviorism. Allopathy is the grossest medicine. That's why it has become scientific, because scientific instrumentation is only capable yet of very gross things. Go deeper.

Acupuncture, the Chinese medicine, enters one layer more. It works on the vital body, the *pranamayakos*. If something goes wrong in the physical body, acupuncture does not touch the physi-cal body at all. It tries to work on the vital body. It tries to work on the bioenergy, the bioplasma. It settles something there, and im-mediately the gross body starts functioning well. If something goes wrong in the vital body, allopathy functions on the body, the gross body. Of course, for allopathy, it is an uphill task. For acupuncture, it is a downhill task. It is easier because the vital body is a little higher than the physical body. If the vital body is set right, the physical body simply follows it because the blueprint exists in the vital body. The physical body is just an implementation of the vital.

Now acupuncture is gaining respect, by and by, because a certain very sensitive photography, Kirlian photography, in Soviet Russia, has come across the seven hundred vital points in the human body as they have always been predicted by acupuncturists for at least five thousand years. They had no instruments to know where the vital points in the body were. But by and by, just through trial and error, through centuries, they discovered seven hundred points. Now Kirlian has also discovered the same seven hundred points with scientific instrumentation. And Kirlian photography has proved one thing: that to try to change the vital through the physical is absurd. It is trying to change the master by changing the servant. It is almost impossible because the master won't listen to the servant. If you want to change the servant, change the master. Immediately, the servant follows. Rather than going and changing each soldier, it is better to change the general. The body has millions of soldiers, cells, simply working under some order, under some commandment. Change the commander, and the whole body pattern changes.

Homeopathy goes still a little deeper. It works on the *mano-mayakos*, the mental body. The founder of homeopathy, Hahnemann, discovered one of the greatest things ever discovered, and that was: the smaller the quantity of the medicine, the deeper it goes. He called the method of making homeopathic medicine 'potentizing'. They go on reducing the quantity of the medicine. He would work in this way: he would take a certain amount of medicine and would mix it with ten times the amount of milk sugar or with water. One quantity of medicine, nine quantities of water; he would mix them. Then he would again take one quantity of this new solution, and would again mix it with nine times more water, or milk sugar. In this way he would go on: again from the new solution he would take one quantity and would mix it with nine times more water. This he would do, and the potency would increase. By and by, the medicine reaches to the atomic level. It becomes so subtle that you cannot believe that it can work; it has almost disappeared. That is what is written on homeopathic medicines, the potency: ten potency, twenty potency, one hundred potency, one thousand potency. The bigger the potency, the smaller is the amount. With ten thousand potency, a millionth of the original medicine has remained, almost none. It has almost disappeared, but then it enters the most deep core of *manomaya*. It enters into your mind body. It goes deeper than acupuncture. It is almost as if you have reached the atomic, or even the sub-atomic level. Then it does not touch your body. Then it does not touch your vital body; it simply enters. It is so subtle and so small that it comes across no barriers. It can simply slip into the *manomayakos*, into the mental body, and from there it starts working. You have found an even bigger authority than the *pranamaya*.

Ayurved, the Indian medicine, is a synthesis of all three. It is one of the most synthetic of medicines.

Hypnotherapy goes still deeper. It touches the *vigyanmayakos*: the fourth body, the body of consciousness. It does not use medicine. It does not use anything. It simply uses suggestion, that's all. It simply puts a suggestion in your mind—call it animal magnetism, mesmerism, hypnosis or whatsoever you like—but it works through the power of thought, not the power of matter. Even homeopathy is still the power of matter in a very subtle quantity. Hypnotherapy gets rid of matter altogether, because howsoever subtle, it is matter. Ten thousand potency, but still, it is a potency of matter. It simply jumps to the thought energy, *vigyanmayakos*: the consciousness body. If your consciousness just accepts a certain idea, it starts functioning.

Hypnotherapy has a great future. It is going to become the future medicine, because if by just changing your thought pattern your mind can be changed, through the mind your vital body and through the vital body your gross body, then why bother with poisons, why bother with gross medicines? Why not work it through thought power? Have you watched any hypnotist working on a medium? If you have not watched, it is worth watching. It will give you a certain insight.

You may have heard, or you may have seen—in India it happens; you must have seen fire-walkers. It is nothing but hypnotherapy. The idea that they are possessed by a certain god or a goddess and no fire can burn them, just this idea is enough. This idea controls and transforms the ordinary functioning of their bodies.

They are prepared: for twenty-four hours they fast. When you are fasting and your whole body is clean, and there is no excreta in it, the bridge between you and the gross drops. For twenty-four hours, they live in a temple or in a mosque, singing, dancing, getting in

tune with God. Then comes the moment when they walk on the fire.
They come dancing, possessed. They come with full trust that the
fire is not going to burn, that's all; there is nothing else. How to
create the trust is the question. Then they dance on the fire, and the
fire does not burn.

It has happened many times that somebody who was just a
spectator became so possessed. Twenty persons walking on fire are
not burned, and somebody would immediately become so
confident: "If these people are walking, then why not I?"; and he
has jumped in, and the fire has not burned. In that sudden moment, a
trust arose. Sometimes it has happened that people who were
prepared, were burned. Sometimes an unprepared spectator
walked on fire and was not burned. What happened?—the people
who were prepared must have carried a doubt. They must have
been thinking whether it was going to happen or not. A subtle
doubt must have remained in the *vigyanmayakos*, in their consciousness. It was not total trust. So they came, but with doubt.
Because of that doubt, the body could not receive the message from
the higher soul. The doubt came in between, and the body continued to function in the ordinary way; it got burned. That's why
all religions insist for trust. Trust is hypnotherapy. Without trust,
you cannot enter into the subtle parts of your being, because a small
doubt, and you are thrown back to the gross. Science works with
doubt. Doubt is a method in science because science works with the
gross. Whether you doubt or not, an allopath is not worried. He does
not ask you to trust in his medicine; he simply gives you medicine.
But a homeopath will ask whether you believe, because without
your belief it will be more difficult for a homeopath to work upon
you. And a hypnotherapist will ask for total surrender. Otherwise,
nothing can be done.

Religion is surrender. Religion is a hypnotherapy. But, there is
still one more body. That is the *anandmayakos*: the bliss body.
Hypnotherapy goes up to the fourth. Meditation goes up to the fifth.
'Meditation'—the very word is beautiful because the root is the
same as 'medicine'. Both come from the same root. Medicine and
meditation are off-shoots of one word: that which heals, that which
makes you healthy and whole is medicine; and on the deepest level,
that is meditation.

Meditation does not even give you suggestions because suggestions are to be given from the outside. Somebody else has to give
you suggestions. Suggestion means that you are dependent upon
somebody. They cannot make you perfectly conscious because the

other will be needed, and a shadow will be cast on your being. Meditation makes you perfectly conscious, without any shadow— absolute light with no darkness. Now even suggestion is thought to be a gross thing. Somebody suggests—that means something comes from the outside, and in the ultimate analysis that which comes from the outside is material. Not only matter, but that which comes from the outside is material. Even a thought is a subtle form of matter. Even hypnotherapy is materialistic.

Meditation drops all props, all supports. That's why to understand meditation is the most difficult thing in the world, because nothing is left—just a pure understanding, a witnessing. That is what this first sutra is.

> *The modifications of the mind are always known by*
> *its lord* ... who is the lord within you? That lord
> has to be found.

> *The modifications of the mind are always known by*
> *its lord, due to the constancy of the Purusa, pure*
> *consciousness.*

In you two things are happening. One is a cyclone of thoughts, emotions, desires—a great whirlwind around you, constantly changing, constantly transforming itself, constantly on the move. It is a process. Behind this process is your witnessing soul—eternal, permanent, not changing at all. It has never changed. It is like the eternal sky: clouds come and go, gather, disperse ... the sky remains untouched, uninfluenced, unimpressed. It remains pure and virgin. That is the lord, the eternal within you.

Mind goes on changing. Just a moment before you had one mind, a moment afterwards you have another mind. Just a few minutes before you were angry, and now you are laughing. Just a moment before you were happy, and now you are sad. Modifications, changes, continuous waves up and down; like a yo-yo you go on. But something in you is eternal: that which goes on witnessing the play, the game. The witnesser is the lord. If you start witnessing, by and by, you will come closer and closer to the lord.

Start witnessing objects. You see a tree. You see the tree, but you are not aware that you are seeing it; then you are not a witness. You see the tree, and at the same time you see that you are seeing; then you are a witness. Consciousness has to become double-arrowed: one arrow going to the tree, another arrow going to your subjectivity.

It is difficult, because when you become aware of yourself you forget the tree, and when you become aware of the tree you forget yourself. But by and by, one learns to balance, just as one learns to balance on a tight-rope. Difficult in the beginning, dangerous, risky, but by and by, one learns the balance. Just go on trying. Wherever you have an opportunity to be a witness, don't miss it, because there is nothing more valuable than witnessing. Doing an act: walking or eating or taking a bath, become a witness also. Let the shower fall on you, but inside you remain alert and see what is happening—the coolness of the water, the tingling sensation all over the body, a certain silence surrounding you, a certain well-being arising in you—but go on becoming a witness. You are feeling happy; just feeling happy is not enough—be a witness. Just go on watching—"I'm feeling happy . . . I'm feeling sad . . . I'm feeling hungry"—go on watching. By and by, you will see that happiness is separate from you, unhappiness also. All that you can witness is separate from you. This is the method of *viveka*, discrimination. All that is separate from you can be witnessed, and all that can be witnessed is separate from you. You cannot witness the witnesser; that is the lord. You cannot go behind the lord; you are the lord. You are the ultimate core of existence.

The mind is not self-illuminating, because it is itself perceptible.

The mind itself can be seen. It can become an object. It can be perceived, so it is not the perceiver. Ordinarily, we think that it is the mind which is seeing the flower. No, you can go beyond the mind and you can see the mind, just as the mind is seeing the flower. The deeper you go, the more you will find that the observer itself becomes the observed. That's why Krishnamurti goes on saying again and again, "The observer is the observed; the perceiver is the perceived." When you go deep, first you see the trees, and the rose and the stars, and you think the mind is witnessing. Then close your eyes. Now, see the impressions in the mind: of roses, stars, trees. Now who is the perceiver? The perceiver has gone a little deeper. Mind itself has become an object.

These five *koshas*, these five seeds, are five stations where the perceiver again and again becomes the perceived. When you move from the gross body, the food body, the *anamayakos*, to the vital body, you immediately see that from the vital body the gross body can be seen as an object. It is outside the vital body. Just as the house is outside you, when you stand in the vital body, your own body is just like a wall around you. Again you move from the vital body to *manomayakos*, the mental body; the same happens. Now, even the vital body is outside you, like a fence around you; and this way it goes on. It goes on to the ultimate point where only the witnesser remains. Then you don't see yourself as, "I am blissful"; you see yourself as a witness of bliss.

The last body is the bliss body. It is the most difficult to separate from because it is very close to the lord. It almost surrounds the lord like a climate. But that too has to be known. Even at that last point when you are ecstatically blissful, then too you have to do the ultimate effort, the last effort of discrimination, and of seeing that the bliss is separate from you.

Then is liberation, *kaivalya*. Then you are left alone—just the witnesser—and everything has been reduced to objects: the body, the mind, the energy. Even the bliss, even the ecstasy, even meditation itself is no more there. When meditation becomes perfect, it is no more a meditation. When the meditator has really achieved the goal, he does not meditate. He cannot meditate because that too is now an activity like walking, eating. He has become separate from everything. That is the difference between *dhyan* and *samadhi*, between meditation and samadhi. Meditation is of the fifth body, the bliss body. It is still a therapy, a medicine. You are still a little ill, ill because you are identifying yourself with something which you are not. All illness is identification, and absolute health is through non-identification. Samadhi is when even meditation has been left behind.

I was reading a book by Edward de Bono. He writes about a very ancient incident that happened in China.

Once, in ancient China, a pagoda, a temple burned down. A strange and appetizing smell led the searchers in the ashes to the roasted body of an unfortunate pig which had got into the blaze, burned in the blaze. Roast pig became a delicacy in China. Accidentally it was discovered because the pagoda burned and a pig was burned in it. But then people thought that it must have something to do with the pagoda, otherwise how could the pig be so delicious? So for centuries in China it continued that whenever they would like to eat a roast pig, they would build a pagoda first, then put a pig inside and burn it down. It was very costly, but it looked very scientific to them. Only after centuries did they become aware that it was foolish. The pig can be roasted without the pagoda. The pagoda is not essential to it.

But this is how the human mind functions, because you become aware of your body first and everything gets associated with it. When you feel a certain well-being, a happiness all around you, of course you feel it is because of the body, because, "I am feeling healthy, no illness, no disease. That's why it is there." Then you try to keep the body young, healthy. Nothing is wrong in it, but well-being comes from somewhere deep within you. Yes, a healthy body is needed, otherwise those deep springs will not be able to be active. A healthy body functions as a vehicle to bring you the well-being from your own innermost core, but the body itself is not the cause.

Let me tell you a few anecdotes on how the mind gets apparently very logical, but deep down comes to very absurd conclusions.

A professor once trained a hundred fleas to jump when he shouted the right command. Once they were responding satisfactorily, he took a pair of scissors and snipped off their legs. As soon as he realized that not one single flea obeyed the command to jump anymore, he announced his findings to the medical world: "I have irrefutable proof, gentlemen, that a flea's ears are situated in its legs."

This has happened many times in the whole history of human thought: legs cut, now they don't jump, they don't listen to the command. Of course, naturally, the ears of the flea are situated in the legs.

Logic can go to very illogical ends. Logic can conclude very illogical conclusions. The body is the most gross part, easily comprehensible; you can catch hold of it, you can train it, you can make it more healthy by giving food, nutrition. You can kill it by starving it. You can do a thousand and one things with the body. It is graspable. Beyond the body starts the world of the elusive.

Scientists are a little afraid to move into the elusive world, because then their criteria don't function well. Then everything goes on becoming dimmer and dimmer. Of course, they stay where light is.

A famous anecdote about Rabia al Adaviya: One evening she was searching for something in the street. Somebody asked, "What are you searching for?" She said, "I have lost my needle." So those people, being kind people, started helping her. "The old woman, poor woman, has lost her needle"; everybody tried to help. But then somebody became aware that a needle is such a small thing: "Exactly where has it fallen? The street is big. If we go on searching it will take millennia." So they asked, "Where exactly has the needle

fallen, so we can search only in that place?" Rabia said, "Don't
ask that, because the needle has fallen inside, in my house." They
all stood up and said, "Have you gone mad! If the needle has fallen
inside, search for it there!" Rabia said, "But there is no light! Here
on the street there is still light. The sun has not yet set. Don't waste
time. Help, because soon the sun will set and the street will be
dark."

In a way, it looks illogical; in another way it seems to be very
logical. That's what science has been doing. The body seems to be
the only lighted part of you; everything else is dark—the deeper you
go, the more dark. The deeper you go, the more direction is lost.
The deeper you go, all that looked clear looks clear no more.
Everything seems to be a tremendous confusion. Better keep to the
lighted part; remain there. Something can be done, because the
body can be manipulated.

But in this way something very valuable is being lost, and
humanity, by and by, has become too focused with the body. And
the body is just your outer shell.

It happened in a prison: Joe was sentenced to twenty years for
his part in a robbery. Shortly after his term of imprisonment
began, he discovered a flea in his hair, and having nothing better to
do, trained it to do tricks. First of all, Joe taught the flea to jump on
command, then gradually the tricks became more and more complex. Every single day of every single week, Joe kept up a routine of
constant practice and calm patience, so that when the day of his
release came he had trained the flea to do tricks which were utterly
unbelievable. As soon as he got outside the prison gates, Joe rushed
to the world's biggest circus. Hurrying into the manager's caravan
Joe produced the flea from his top pocket and placed it on the table,
"Just look at this," said Joe to the manager. "Yes," said the
manager, as he slammed a large heavy ashtray down on the flea.
"Nuisances, are they not?"

He killed the flea, and now there is no way for that poor Joe to
prove that he had trained the flea to do almost miraculous things,
unbelievable things. Now there is no way to prove it.

That's what gross thinking about humanity has done: it has
killed the inner mystery. It has made people so addicted with the
body that they have forgotten their inner world. Now even to prove
it has become difficult. People like Buddha and Jesus and Krishna
look insane. There are books in the English language and in other
Western languages proving Jesus to be neurotic. Of course, if you
have not known anything of the inner world, he looks neurotic. He

is neurotic if you don't know anything about the inner world. Then
he seems to be like a madman because sometimes he talks to God,
and he declares that he receives the answers also. And you have lost
all contact with the inner world, so what is the difference between
a madman and him? A madman also listens to voices. You can see;
go to the madhouse and you can see mad people sitting alone and
talking so enchantedly, as if somebody is present there. What is the
difference? When in the Garden of Gethsemane Jesus prayed, raised
his hands towards the sky and started talking to God, what is the
difference? There seems to be nobody there. Jesus is as mad as the
madman. When on the cross he started crying and saying things to
God, what is the difference? Because many thousands of people had
gathered there; they could not see anybody there. And Jesus said,
"Father, forgive these people, because they don't know what they
are doing." He is mad. To whom was he talking? He had gone out
of his senses. By and by, if your innermost world is crippled and
you have lost contact with it, you cannot believe in Jesus, Krishna,
Buddha, or Patanjali. What are they talking about? These people
are dreaming. And you, very clever people, go on talking about your
dreaming in a very scientific way.

Many mad people are very, very logical. If you listen to mad
people, you will be surprised. They are very argumentative, very
rational; and up to a certain extent you will be almost convinced by
them.

I have heard about one man who went to see some relative who
was in a madhouse. In the same cell there was another inmate, and
the other man looked so gentlemanly, so graceful, and was sitting
with such dignity reading a newspaper, that this visitor asked,
"You don't look mad at all." He talked with that man and he was
perfectly logical, absolutely normal. The visitor was surprised:
"Why have you been kept?" He said, "Because of my relatives; they
wanted to throw me in here because they want to grab all the
money that I have, and that is the only way: either to kill me, or to
throw me into a madhouse. And I also agreed. This is better. At
least I am alive. Otherwise, they would have killed me. I have such
a lot of money."

And everything was so logical and normal that the visitor said,
"You don't be worried. I know the governor, and I will go to him
and tell everything." The madman said, "Please, if you can do
something, do it." When the visitor was just leaving the room,
suddenly the madman jumped and hit him hard on the head. The
visitor said, "What are you doing?" He said, "Just to remind you
. . . don't forget to go to the governor. Now you will not forget."

Everything was logical somewhere, but how to differentiate between a madman and a mystic? Because everything seems to be logical in a mystic also, to a certain extent. Then suddenly, he is talking of something which you have not ever experienced. Then you become afraid, and to protect yourself from the fear, you start rationalizing your fear.

It is impossible for the mind to know itself and any
other object at the same time.

These sutras are all about witnessing. Patanjali is saying, step by step, that it is impossible for the mind to do two things: to be perceived and to be the perceiver. Either it can be the perceiver or it can be the perceived. So when you can witness your mind, that proves absolutely that the mind is not the perceiver. You are the perceiver. You are not the body; you are not even the mind. The whole emphasis is: how to help you to discriminate from that which you are not.

If it were assumed that a second mind illuminates
the first, cognition of cognition would have to be
assumed, and a confusion of memories.

But there have been philosophers who say that there is no need to assume a witness; we can assume another mind: mind one is perceived by mind two. That's what psychologists will also agree to, because why bring something absolutely unknown into account?—mind is observed by mind itself, by a subtle mind. But Patanjali gives a very logical refutation of this attitude. He says, "If you assume that mind one is perceived by mind two, then who perceives mind two? Then mind three; then who perceives mind three?" He says, "Then this will create confusion. It will be an infinite regress. Then you can go on, ad absurdum; and again, even if you say 'the mind one thousand', the problem remains the same. Then you have to again assume a mind behind mine one thousand: one thousand and one—and this will go on and on.

No, one has to understand something absolutely inside, behind which there is nothing. Otherwise there is a confusion of memories, otherwise, a chaos. Body, mind, and the witnesser: the witnesser is absolute. But who perceives the witnesser? Who knows the witnesser? And then we come to one of the most important hypotheses of yoga.

Knowledge of its own nature through self-cognition
is obtained when consciousness assumes that form
in which it does not pass from place to place.

Yoga believes that the witness is a self-illuminating phenomenon. It is just like a light. You have a small candle in your
room—the candle illuminates the room, the furniture, the walls, the
painting on the wall. Who illuminates the candle? You don't need
another candle to find this candle; the candle is self-illuminating. It
illuminates other things, and simultaneously it illuminates itself.
Svabuddhi-samvedanam: innermost consciousness is self-illuminating. It is of the nature of light. The sun illuminates everything
in the solar system—at the same time it illuminates itself. The
witnesser witnesses everything that goes on around in the five seeds
and in the world, and at the same time it illuminates itself. This
seems to be perfectly logical. Somewhere, we have to come to the
rock bottom. Otherwise, we go on and on—and that will not help,
and the problem remains the same.

Knowledge of its own. nature through
*self-cognition—*svabuddhi-samvedanam—*is*
obtained when consciousness assumes that form in
which it does not pass from place to place.

When your inner consciousness has come to a moment of no
movement, when it has become deeply centered and rooted, when
it is unwavering, when it has become a constant flame of awareness, then it illuminates itself.

When the mind is colored by the knower and the
known, it is all-apprehending.

The mind is just between you and the world. The mind is the
bridge between you and the world, between the witnesser and the
witnessed. The mind is a bridge, and if the mind is colored by
things, and also by the witness, it becomes all-comprehending. It
becomes a tremendous instrument of knowledge. But two types of
coloring are needed; one: it should be colored by the things it sees,
and, it should be colored by the witnesser. The witnesser should
pour down its energy into the mind; then only can the mind know
things.
For example: a scientist is working. He has dissected the body of

a man and he is looking very minutely, as minutely as scientific instruments make available. He is searching for the soul, and he cannot find any soul, just matter, matter. At the most, he can find something belonging to the world of physics or to the world of chemistry, but nothing belonging to the world of consciousness. And he comes out of the lab, and he says, "There is no consciousness." Now, he has missed one thing. Who was looking in the dead body? He has completely forgotten himself. The scientist is watching the object but is completely oblivious of his own being. The scientist is trying to find consciousness outside, but has forgotten completely that the one who is trying is consciousness. The seeker is the sought. He has become too much focused on the object, and the subject is forgotten.

Science is too focused on the object, and so-called religions are too focused on the subject. But yoga says, "There is no need to become lopsided. Remember the world is there, and also remember that you are." Let your remembrance be total and whole, of the object and the subject both. When your mind is infused with your consciousness, and also infused with the objective world, there happens apprehension.

And Patanjali says, *When the mind is colored by the knower and the known, it is all-apprehending.*

It can know all that can be known. It can know everything that can be known. Then nothing is hidden from that mind. A religious mind—let us call him an introvert—by and by, knows only his subjectivity and starts saying that the world is illusion, *maya*, a dream, made of the same stuff as dreams are. A scientist who is too focused on objects starts believing in the objective world and says that only the material exists; consciousness is just poetry, a talk of the dreamers: good, romantic, but not real. The scientist says that consciousness is illusory. The extrovert says that consciousness is illusory; the introvert says that the world is illusory.

But yoga is the supreme science. Patanjali says, "Both are real." Reality has two sides to it: the outside and the inside. And remember, how can the inside happen, how can it exist without an outside? Can you conceive that only the inside exists and the outside is illusory? If the outside is illusory, the inside will become illusory automatically. If the inside of your house is real, and the outside of the house is unreal, where will you demarcate? Where does the reality stop and illusion start? And how can an outside which is illusory have a real inside? An unreal body will have an unreal mind; an unreal mind will have an unreal consciousness. A real consciousness needs a real mind; a real mind needs a real body; a real body needs a real world.

Yoga does not deny anything. Yoga is absolutely pragmatic, empirical. It is more scientific than science, and more religious than religions, because it makes the greater synthesis of the inner and the outer.

Though variegated by innumerable desires, the mind acts for another, for it acts in association.

The mind goes on working, but it is not working for itself. It has a managerial post; the master is hidden behind. It cooperates with the master. Now, this has to be deeply understood.

If the mind cooperates with the master, you are healthy and whole. If the mind goes astray, against the master, you are unhealthy and ill. If the servant follows the master like a shadow, everything is okay. If the master says, "Go to the left," and the servant goes to the right, then something has gone wrong. If you want your body to run and the body says, "I cannot run," then you are paralyzed. If you want to do something and the body and the mind say, "No," or, they go on doing something which you don't want to do, then you are in great confusion. This is how humanity is.

Yoga has this as the goal: that your mind should function according to your lord, the innermost soul. Your body should function according to the mind, and you should create a world around you which is in cooperation. When everything is in cooperation—the lower is always in cooperation with the higher, and the higher is in cooperation with the highest, and the highest is in cooperation with the utterly ultimate—then you have a life of harmony. Then you are a *yogin*. Then you become one, but not in the sense that only one exists: now you have become one in the sense of unison. You have become one in the sense of an orchestra—many instruments, but the music is one; many bodies, millions of objects, desires, ambitions, mood, ups and downs, failures and successes, a great variety, but everything in unison, in harmony. You have become an orchestra. Everything is cooperating with everything else, and everything finally is cooperating with the very center of your being.

That's why in India we have called sannyasins *swamis*. 'Swami'

means: the lord. You become a swami only when you have attained
to this harmony that Patanjali is talking about. Patanjali is not
against anything whatsoever. He is in favor of harmony. He's
against discord. He is not against anything: he's not against the
body, he's not an anti-body man; he's not against the world, he's
not anti-life; he absorbs everything. And through that absorption he
creates a higher synthesis. And the ultimate synthesis is when
everything is in cooperation, when there is not even a single jarring
note.

I have heard an anecdote: The baby baboon was five years old
but had not spoken a word since birth. Its parents were convinced
that their offspring was dumb until one night when the little
baboon was eating a banana. It suddenly looked up at its mother
and spoke clearly: "What is the idea of feeding me a rotten
banana?" The mother baboon was overjoyed and asked her baby
why he had never spoken before. "Well," said the little baboon,
"the food has been okay up to now."

If you are in a harmony, you will not complain about the world.
You will not complain about anything. The complaining mind is
simply indicative that things are not in harmony inside. When
everything is in harmony, then there is no complaint. Now, you go
to your so-called saints: everybody is complaining—complaining of
the world, complaining of desires, complaining of the body, complaining of this and that. Everybody lives in complaints; something
is jarring. A perfect man is one who has no complaints. That man is
a God-man who has accepted everything, absorbed everything and
become a cosmos, is no more a chaos.

Another anecdote: The sweet little old lady was proud of the way
she had trained her talking parrot, and was showing him off to the
vicar. "If you pull his left leg, he says the Lord's Prayer, and if you
pull his right leg, he repeats the Psalms," she explained.

"What if you pull both legs at once?" asked the vicar.

"I would fall flat on my behind, you stupid old coot!" retorted
the parrot.

And this is what has happened to man. If you pull one leg it is
okay; if you pull the other leg, that too is okay; but if you pull both
legs, everything is bound to topple down. That's what has happened to man. His whole being has been pulled down. Religions
have been trying to pull his body. They are much too afraid of the
body, too guilty. They have been continuously trying to destroy and
poison the body. They would like you to be like ghosts, without
bodies. Their idea is that body is intrinsically wrong, that body is

the body of sin. So you should be like spirits—without bodies, disembodied.

Now the materialists—the communists, the Marxists, the scientists—have been trying the other way. They have been trying to pull the other leg. They say that there is nothing like consciousness; there is no self. It is just a combination of physical and chemical things that you are. You should be a body, nothing else. Now, both together have pulled both legs, and the whole man has become a miserable thing, a disease, a dichotomy.

Patanjali says, "Accept everything, use it, be creative about it; don't negate." Negation is not his way, but affirmation. That's why Patanjali has worked so much on the body, on food, on yoga *asanas*, on *pranayam*. These are all efforts to create the harmony: right food for the body, right posture for the body; rhythmic breathing for the vital body. More *prana*, more vitality has to be absorbed. Ways and means have to be found so that you are not always lacking in energy, but overflowing.

With mind also, *pratyahar;* the mind is a bridge: you can go outside on the bridge, you can move on the same bridge and go inside. When you go outside, objects, desires, predominate you. When you go inside, desirelessness, awareness, witnessing, predominate over you; but the bridge is the same. It has to be used; it is not to be thrown and broken. It has not to be destroyed because it is the same bridge by which you have come into the world, and by which you have to go back again into the inner nature, and so on and so forth.

Patanjali goes on using everything. His religion is not one of fear, but of understanding. His religion is not for God and against the world. His religion is for God through the world, because God and the world are not two. The world is God's creation. The world is His creativity, His expression; the world is His poetry. If you are against the poetry, how can you be in favor of the poet? In condemning the poetry, you have already condemned the poet. Of course, poetry is not the goal; you should seek the poet also. But on the way you can enjoy the poetry; nothing is wrong in it.

A methodist minister was on a flight to America when the stewardess asked if he would like a drink from the bar. "At what height are we flying?" he asked. When told that it was thirty thousand feet, he replied, "I would rather not . . . too near headquarters."

Fear—continuously, religious people are obsessed by fear. But fear cannot give you a grace, cannot give you a dignity. Fear cripples, paralyzes, corrupts. Because of fear religion has become almost a disease. It makes you abnormal. It does not make you healthy, it makes you more and more afraid to live: hell is there, and whatsoever you do it seems to be that you are doing something wrong. You love and it is wrong; you enjoy and it is wrong. Happiness has become associated with guilt. Only wrong people seem to be happy. The good people are always serious and never happy. If you want to go to heaven you have to be serious and unhappy and sad and miserable. You have to be austere. If you want to go to hell, be happy and dance and enjoy. But remember, Omar Khayyam says somewhere, "I am always worried about one thing: if all these unhappy people are going to heaven, what will they do there? They cannot dance, they cannot sing, they cannot drink, they cannot enjoy, they cannot love. The whole opportunity will be wasted on these foolish people. People who could enjoy are thrown into hell. In fact, they should be in heaven. It seems more logical." Omar Khayyam says, "If you really want to go to heaven, live a heavenly life here, so that you are ready."

Patanjali would like you to radiate with life, to throb with the unknown. He is not against anything. If you are in love he says, "Make your love a little more deep." There are greater treasures waiting for you. These treasures are good; these trees, these flowers, are good. Then man, woman, they are good and beautiful, because somehow, howsoever far away, God has come to you through them. Maybe there are many screens. When you meet a man or a woman, there are many screens and sheets, but still the light is of God. It may be passing through many barriers, it may be distorted, but still, the light is of God.

Patanjali says, "Don't be against this world. Rather, search through this world. Find a way so that you can come to the original source of light, the pure, the virgin light."

There are people who live only for food, and there are people who go against food—both are wrong. Jesus says, "Man cannot live by bread alone"—true, perfectly true—but can man live without bread? That has to be remembered. Man cannot live by bread alone, right; but man also cannot live without bread.

I was reading a small anecdote.

The woman bought a budgerigar from the pet shop on the assurance that it would talk. Two weeks later she was back to complain. "Buy a little bell for it to play with," suggested the pet shop owner. "That often helps to get them talking." The woman bought the bell and went off. A week later she was back to say the bird had still not uttered a word. The shop owner suggested that she buy a mirror, which was a sure-fire way of encouraging budgies to talk. She took the mirror and went away, only to return in another three days. This time the shop owner sold her a small plastic bird which he suggested would give the bird something to talk to. Another week passed and the woman came in to inform the shop owner that the bird had now died.

"Did he die without ever speaking?" asked the shop owner.

"Ah, no," replied the woman. "It said one thing shortly before it passed away."

"What was that?"

"Food! For Pete's sake, give me food!"

One has to be very, very alert, otherwise one can move to opposite polarities very easily. Mind is an extremist. This is my observation: people who have lived only for food, when they get frustrated with their life-style, start fasting. Immediately, they move to the other extreme. I have never come across a faster, a fanatic about fasting, who has not previously been a fanatic about food. They are the same people. People who are too much in sexuality start becoming celibate. People who are very miserly start renouncing everything. This is how the mind moves from one extreme to another.

Patanjali would like you to balance your life, to bring an equilibrium. Just in the middle somewhere, where you are not mad after food and you are not mad against food, where you are not mad after women or men and you are not mad against them; you are simply balanced, a tranquility.

A psychiatrist says that we are a little strange in our behavior. We all are a little strange in our behavior. Another way of saying this is: I am original, you are eccentric, he is nuts. When you do the same thing you think you are original, when your friend is doing the same thing you think he is eccentric, and when your enemy is doing the same thing you think he is nuts. Remember, this egoistic way of thinking will destroy all the opportunities for growth. Be very objective about yourself. There is a strain of insanity in everybody, because humanity has been insane for millennia. There is a strain of neurosis in everybody, because civilization has not yet come to a point where it can allow the full functioning of the human being. It has been repressive. So watch: if you are neurotic you will eat too much. You can move to the other extreme—you can stop eating completely—but your neurosis remains the same. Now, the neurosis is against food. And don't think that you are doing great spiritual work, very original work.

Once Veena brought a boy to me. In fact, that is how she got caught with me. She had come with some other boy who was almost neurotic. He had come to ask me, "Can man live on water alone?" He wanted to live on water alone. And he was very thin, and almost dying and pale. When I said, "Don't be foolish," he was not happy. He said, "You just give me some address, some people who can help me, because I want to live only on water. Everything is impure—just pure water."

These people are neurotic. You can find them all over India: in monasteries, in ashrams. Out of a hundred people you will find ninety-five neurotic. And you cannot call them mad because they are doing yoga asanas, fasting, prayer, this and that. But their neurosis can be seen immediately, what I call neurosis. Any extremism is neurotic. To be balanced is to be healthy; to be unbalanced is to be neurotic. Wherever you find any unbalance within yourself or in somebody else, beware. Otherwise, you will miss the ultimate unison. Lopsided, unbalanced, you cannot create the orchestra that Patanjali is trying to give you a glimpse of.

> *The modifications of the mind are always known by its lord, due to the constancy of the Purusa, pure consciousness.*
>
> *Sada jnatas citta-vritayas tat-prabhu purusasyaparinamitvat.*

Tat-prabhu, the lord has to be found. He's hiding in you; you have to seek him. Whatsoever you are, he's present. Whatsoever you do, he's the doer. Whatsoever you see, he's the seer. Even whatsoever you desire, it is he who has desired it. Layer upon layer, like an onion, you have to peel yourself. But peel yourself not in a rage, but in love. Peel yourself very cautiously, carefully, because it is God you are peeling. Peel very prayerfully. Don't become a masochist. Don't start creating suffering for yourself. Don't enjoy suffering. If you start enjoying suffering and you become a masochist, you are going on a suicidal trip. You will destroy yourself. One has to be very, very cautious, careful and creative. You are moving on holy ground.

When Moses reached to the top of the mountain where he encountered God, what did he see? He saw in a bush, a flame, a fire, and he heard a voice: "Leave your shoes off, because it is holy ground you are walking on." But wherever you are walking, you are walking on holy ground. When you touch your body, you are touching something holy. When you eat something, you are eating something holy; *annambrahma:* food is God. When you love somebody, you are loving the divine, because it is He all around, in millions of forms. It is He who is expressing.

Keep this always in mind so that no neurosis can take possession of you. Remain balanced and tranquil, just walk the path in the middle, and you will never be lost, you will never be unbalanced, lopsided.

Yoga is balance. Yoga has to be a balance because it is going to be the path to the ultimate unity, the ultimate harmony of all that is.

CHAPTER EIGHT
May 8, 1976

TRUST IS UNADDRESSED

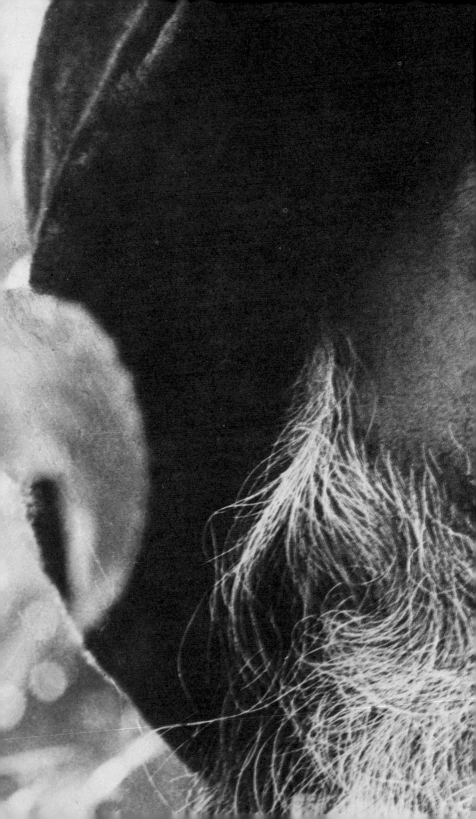

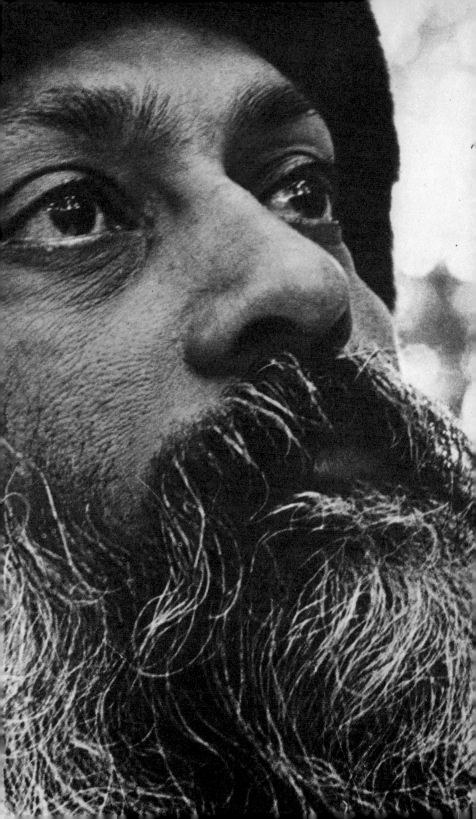

The first question:

In one of your lectures something has hit me hard. It is the contradiction between trusting myself and trusting you. There is a part of me that says: if I trust my own self and follow my own self, then I have surrendered and said yes to you. But I am not sure whether that is just a rationalization I have created for myself.

THE MIND IS VERY CUNNING, and that has to be constantly remembered. This is what I have been saying to you: that if you trust yourself, you will trust me. Or, from the other side, if you trust me you will naturally trust yourself. The contradiction does not exist. The contradiction arises because of the mind. If you trust yourself you trust all, because you trust life. You trust even those who will deceive you, but that is irrelevant. That is their problem; it is not your problem. Whether they deceive you or they don't deceive you, it has nothing to do with your trust. If you say, "My trust exists only with a condition that nobody tries to deceive me," then your trust cannot exist because every possibility will create a certain hesitation in you: "Who knows?—the person may be going to deceive me." How can you see the future? The deception will happen in the future, if it happens, or if it does not happen, that too is in the future—and trust has to be here-now.

And sometimes a very good man can deceive you. A saint can become a sinner at any moment. And sometimes a very bad man can be very deeply trustworthy. After all, sinners become saints. But that is in the future, and if you make a condition for your trust, then you cannot trust. Trust is unconditional. It simply says that, "I have that quality which trusts. Now, it is irrelevant what happens to my trust—whether it is respected or not, whether it is deceived or not. That is not the point at all." Trust has nothing to do with the object of trust, it has something to do with your inner quality: can you trust? If you can trust, of course the first trust will happen about yourself—you trust yourself. The first thing has to happen at the deepest core of your being. If you don't trust yourself then everything is very far away. Then I am very far away from you.

How can you trust me? You have not trusted even yourself who is so close. And how can you trust your trust about me if you don't trust yourself? If you don't trust yourself, whatsoever you do, a deep mistrust will continue as an undercurrent. If you trust yourself, you trust the whole life—not only me, because why only me? Trust is all-inclusive. Trust means: trust in life, the whole that surrounds you; the whole out of which you have come, and the whole into which one day you will dissolve.

Trust simply means that you have understood the neurosis of doubt, that you have understood the misery of doubt, that you have understood the hell that doubt creates. You have known doubt and by knowing it you have dropped it. When doubt disappears, there is trust. It is something of a transformation within you, your attitude, approach. Trust knows no contradiction.

The questioner asks, "It is the contradiction between trusting myself and trusting you." If that is the contradiction, then trust yourself. If you can trust yourself nothing else is needed. Then you are deeply rooted in your trust, and when a tree is deeply rooted in the earth, it goes on spreading its branches into the unknown sky. When it is rooted in the earth, it can trust the sky. When the tree is not rooted in the earth, then it cannot trust the sky; then it is always afraid: afraid of the storm, afraid of the rains, afraid of the sun, afraid of the wind, afraid of everything. The fear is coming from the roots. The tree knows that she is not rooted perfectly. Any slight accident, and she will be gone. She is already gone. Such a life, unrooted, uncentered, is not a life at all. It is just a slow, long suicide. So if you trust yourself, forget all about me. There is no need even to raise the question. But you know and I know that you don't trust yourself.

The mind is creating a very cunning device. The mind is saying, "Don't trust anybody, trust yourself"; and you cannot trust yourself. That's why you are here. Otherwise why would you be here? One who trusts himself need not go anywhere, need not go to any Master, need not go to learn anywhere. Life is coming to you in millions of ways; there is no need to go anywhere.

Wherever you are truth will happen, but you don't trust yourself. And when I say, "Trust me," that is only a device to help you trust. You cannot trust yourself?—okay; trust me. Maybe trusting me will give you a taste of trust; then you can trust yourself.

The Master is nothing but a long way to come to yourself, because you cannot come through the shortest way. You have to follow a little longer route. But via the Master, you come to yourself. If you are stuck with me then I am your enemy, then I have not been a help to you. Then I don't love you, then I don't have any compassion for you. If I have any compassion, then by and by, I will turn you back towards yourself. That's what I go on saying: "If you meet a Buddha on the way, kill him!" If you start clinging to me, drop me immediately. Kill me, forget all about me. But your mind will say, "When there is so much fear of clinging, it is better never to start the journey." Then you remain in self distrust. I'm simply giving you an opportunity to have a taste of trust.

Listening to me when I say don't cling to the Master, your ego starts feeling very good. It says, "Perfectly true. Why should I trust anybody? Why should I surrender to anybody? Exactly, this is the right thing!" That's what has happened to J. Krishnamurti's disciples. For forty, fifty years he has been teaching, and there are many who have listened their whole lives to him, and nothing has happened—because he goes on insisting that there is no Master, no disciple. He goes on throwing you upon yourself. Even before you have a taste of trust, he goes on throwing you upon yourself. Before you start clinging he's alert, very alert. He will not allow you to approach near him. This is one extreme. Your ego feels very good that you don't have any Master, that you don't have to surrender to anybody. You?—and surrendering? It does not look good; looks like humiliation. You feel very good. With Krishnamurti, all sorts of egoists have gathered together around him. If you want to find the most cultured egoists, then you will find them around Krishnamurti. They are very cultured, sophisticated, very intellectual, very cunning and clever, logical, rationalizers, but nothing has happened to them. Many of them come to me and they say, "We know, we understand, but our understanding has remained intellectual. Nothing has happened. We have not been transformed, so what is the point?" Krishnamurti says don't cling to him, but you are clinging to yourself. If there is any choice to be made, better to cling to Krishnamurti than clinging to yourself. At least you are clinging to a better person.

Then there is another extreme. There are gurus who insist that you should cling to them. Surrender seems to be the end, not the means. They say, "Remain completely with me. Never allow any movement back to your home." That too seems to be dangerous, because then you are always on the path and never reach the goal—because the goal is you. I can become a path; Krishnamurti won't allow you to make him a path. Then there are others who won't allow you to become the goal. They say, "Go on travelling, go on travelling." You remain always on the pilgrimage and you never arrive—because arrival has to be at your innermost core of being. I cannot be your arrival. How can I be your arrival? One day or other you have to make me a departure.

I'm neither in agreement with Krishnamurti, nor with the other extremists. I say: use me as a path, but *as a path* remember. And if I start becoming a goal, kill me immediately, drop me immediately—because now the medicine is becoming like a disease. Medicine has to be used and forgotten. You should not carry the bottles and the prescription continuously with you. It was a means, instrumental; now you are healthy, drop it, forget all about it. Be thankful to it, be grateful to it, but there is no need to carry it.

Buddha has said that five fools crossed a river, then they all started thinking—fools are always philosophers, and the vice versa is also true—they started thinking, "What to do? This boat has helped us so tremendously, otherwise we would have died on the other side. It was wild, and night was coming, and there were wild animals and robbers, and anything could have happened. This boat has saved us. We should be grateful always and always for this boat, towards this boat." Then one fool suggested, "Yes, that's right. Now we should carry the boat on our heads because this boat has to be worshipped." So they started carrying the boat towards the town on their heads. Many people asked, "What are you doing? We have seen people sitting in a boat; we have never seen a boat sitting on people. What has happened?" They said, "You don't know. This boat has saved our lives. Now we cannot forget, and for our whole lives we are going to carry this boat on our heads." Now, this boat killed them completely. It would have been better to be left on the other side of the river. It would have been better to be killed by the wild animals rather than carry this boat forever and ever. This was an endless misery. On the other side of the river, at least within a second, things would have happened. Now for years together they would carry the load, the burden, the boredom. And the more they carry, the more they will become accustomed to the load. Without the load they will not feel good; they will feel uncomfortable. And now they will not be able to do anything, because how to do anything else? Carrying the boat will be so continuously absorbing that they will become almost incapable of doing anything.

That's what has happened to many religious people: they have become incapable of doing anything; they are simply carrying their boat. Go and see the Jain monasteries, Catholic monasteries,

Buddhist monasteries—what are people doing? They are just doing religion; the whole life has been dropped. They are just praying, or just meditating. What are they doing? Life is not enriched by them. They are not creative. They are a curse, they are not a blessing. Life does not become more beautiful because of them. They are not helping in any way. But they are very serious people, and they look continuously engaged; for twenty-four hours they are engaged. They are carrying a boat on their heads. Their ritual is their boat.

Remember: come to me, trust me. Just learn what trust is. Come to my garden and listen to the wind passing through the trees, just to go back home and create a garden of your own. Come to these flowers, these singing birds; have a deep experience of them, then go back. Then create your own world. Just through my window, have a glimpse. Let me flash like lightning before you so you can see the whole of life—but it is going to be just a glimpse.

No need to cling to me, because then, when will you make your own house, and when will you make your own garden, and when will your own flowers flower, and when will your own birds of the heart sing? No, then you will carry the boat that helped you to the other shore. But then that other shore is already destroyed because you will be carrying your boat on your heads. How will you dance on the other shore? How will you celebrate? That boat will be a constant imprisonment.

When I tell you to trust me, I am simply saying that a certain climate has happened to me: have a glimpse of it. Come, let that climate surround you also. Let me vibrate in your heart; let me pulsate around you; let me throb in the deepest core of your being; let me resound in you. I am singing a song here—let it be echoed so that you can know that, "Yes, the song is possible." Buddha is gone, Jesus is not here; it's natural. Listening to Jesus is not possible for you. You can read the Bible; it simply depicts something that happened somewhere in time, but you cannot believe it. It may be just a myth, a story. Buddha may be just of a poetic imagination; poets may have created him. Who knows?—because in life you don't come across such men. Unless you come across a religious man, religion will remain somewhere like a dream. It will never become a reality. If you come across a man who has tasted of truth, who has lived in a different world and in a different dimension, to whom God has happened and to whom God is not just a theory, but a fact like breathing, then trust him, go into him. Then don't hesitate; then take courage. Then be a little bold. Then don't be a coward and don't go on slinking outside the door; enter the temple. Of course, this temple is not going to become an abode for you. You will have to create your own temple—because God can be worshipped only when you have created your own temple. In a borrowed temple, God cannot be worshipped. God is a creator and respects only creativity. And the basic creativity is to create a temple of your own. No, borrowed temples won't do. But, how to create a temple?

In the first place, it is almost impossible to believe that temples have ever existed. Jesus' existence remains doubtful; Buddha looks like a myth, not like history; Krishna is even more in the world of dreams. The farther back you go in history, the more and more things fade into mythologies. No signature is left on reality.

When I say trust me, I simply mean: don't stand outside. If you have come so close to me, come a little more close. If you have come, then come in. Then let my climate surround you. That will become an existential experience to you. Looking into my eyes, entering into my heart, it will become impossible for you then to distrust Jesus. It will be impossible for you then to say that Buddha is just a myth. But still, I will go on saying that if Buddha comes, meets you on the path, kill him.

Come through me, but don't stay there. Have the experience and go on your way. If the experience is lost again in memories and fades out, come again to me while I'm available here. Have another dip, but remember continuously that you have to create something of your own. Only then can you live in it. I can be a holiday, at the most, from your ordinary life, but I cannot become your life. You will have to change your life.

Now, the mind is very cunning. If I say trust me, the mind feels it is difficult. Trusting somebody else is very ego-destroying. If I say just trust yourself, the mind feels very good. But just by feeling good, nothing happens. I say to you, trust yourself. If it is possible, there is no need to trust me; if it is not possible, then try the other. Mind is always in search through everything to somehow make itself more strengthened.

I will tell you one anecdote.

A country dweller moved to the big city, and every Sunday for about six months, he attended a different church in an endeavor to find a congenial congregation. Finally, one Sunday morning, he entered a church just as the congregation recited with the minister, "We have left undone those things which we ought to have done, and we have done those things which we ought not to have done." He sat down with a sigh of relief and satisfaction, murmuring to himself, "At last I have found my lot."

You are just trying to find something which does not disturb you. On the contrary, it strengthens your old mind. It strengthens you as you are. That is the whole effort of the mind: to perpetuate itself. You will have to be mindful about it. The mind has the tendency to hear not that which is said, but that which it wants to hear.

Harry had married his elderly, ugly wife only for her money. Of course, he found plenty of ways to spend it, like the present safari trek through the African jungle. When a huge alligator slipped out of the marshes, grabbed his wife between its teeth and started to pull her away, Harry did not move a muscle. "Quick! Shoot it!! Shoot it!" screamed his unfortunate wife. Harry shrugged, "I would love to, dear, but I haven't any film in my camera."

The mind has the tendency to hear what it wants to hear. Never think that you are hearing me. You go on manipulating it in many ways. When something enters into your head, you don't listen to it directly. First, you mix it with your ideas; you change here and there. A few things you drop, a few things you add. Then of course it starts suiting you, by and by, and you convince yourself that that is what was said to you.

A tramp collapsed on a London street during a very hot spell, and immediately a crowd gathered around him.

"Give the poor fellow a drop of whisky," said an old lady.

"Give him some air," said a man.

"Give him some whisky," said the old lady again.

"Take him to the hospital," said another gent.

"Give him some whisky," said the old dear once again.

The conversation went on like this till the tramp sat up and yelled, "Will you all belt up and listen to the old lady!"

Even when you are unconscious, you can listen to that which you want to listen to; and even when you are conscious you are not listening to that which is being said to you.

One beggar comes here to listen to me. That beggar approached a fellow in the main street and said, "Give me a few *annas* for a cup of coffee." The man said, "But I gave you eight *annas* only ten minutes ago." The tramp said, "Oh, stop living in the past." Continuously I am teaching you to stop living in the past—perfectly true.

Remember, your mind continuously is playing tricks on you. There is no contradiction; contradiction is created by you.

Now, I will read the remaining part of the question—see the emphasis. "There is a part of me that says if I trust my own self and follow my own self, then I have surrendered and said yes to you."

But this is only a part; and what about the remaining? If you trust this part, the remaining mind will say, "What are you doing?" That's how the doubt arises. If you listen to the remaining part, this part will go on creating doubts. This is how the mind moves— always in a dichotomy. It divides itself against itself, and it goes on playing the game of hide and seek. So whatsoever you do, frustration comes—whatsoever. But the frustration is bound to come. If you trust me, one part of your mind will go on saying, "What are you doing?" I have always been telling you, just trust yourself. If you don't trust me and trust yourself, the other part of the mind will continuously be frustrating. It will say, "What are you doing? Trust him. Surrender." Now, look at the dichotomy of the mind.

If you can see this constant division of the mind which is never able to come to a total decision, then by and by, a different type of consciousness will arise in you which can decide totally. That is not of the mind. That's why I say that surrender is not of the mind. Trust is not of the mind. Mind *cannot* trust. Distrust is very intrinsic to mind; it is inbuilt. Mind exists on distrust, on doubt. When you are in too much doubt, you see too much mentation around inside, moving. Mind gets in too much activity. But when you trust, there is nothing for the mind to do. Have you watched it? When you say, "No!" you throw a rock into the silent pool of your consciousness; millions of ripples arise. When you say, "Yes" you are not throwing any rock. At the most, you may be floating a rose flower in the lake. Without any ripple, the flower floats. That's why people find it very difficult to say yes, and find it very easy to say no. 'No' is always just ready. Even before you have heard, the no is ready.

I was staying with Mulla Nasrudin once. I heard the wife saying to Nasrudin, "Nasrudin, just go and see what the boy is doing, and stop him."

She does not know what the boy is doing: "Just go and see what the boy is doing, and stop him." Whatsoever it is, is not the point; but stopping, saying no. Denying comes easy; it enhances the ego. The ego feeds on no; the mind feeds on doubt, suspicion, distrust. You cannot trust me through the mind. You will have to see the dichotomy of the mind—the constant duel, the constant debate inside the mind. One part is always functioning as the opposition.

The mind never comes to a decision. There are always a few fragments of the mind as dissenters. They wait for their opportunity, and they will frustrate you.

Then what is trust? How can you trust? You have to understand the mind. By understanding the mind and the constant duality in it, by witnessing it, you become separate from the mind. And in that separation arises trust, and that trust knows no division between me and you. That trust knows no division between you and life. That trust is simply trust. It is unaddressed trust, not addressed to anybody—because if you trust me, you will immediately distrust somebody. Whenever you trust somebody, immediately, on the other end, you will be mistrusting somebody else. If you believe in the Koran, you cannot believe in Buddha. If you trust in Jesus, you cannot trust in Buddha. What type of trust is this? It is of no worth.

Trust is unaddressed. It is neither addressed to Christ, nor to Buddha. It's simple trust. You simply trust because you enjoy trusting. You simply trust, and you enjoy trusting so much that even when you are deceived, you enjoy. You enjoy that you could trust even when there was every possibility of deception, that the deception could not destroy your trust, that your trust was greater, that the deceiver could not corrupt you. He may have taken your money, he may have taken your prestige, he may have robbed you completely, but you will enjoy. And you will feel tremendously happy and blissful that he could not corrupt your trust; you still trust him. And if he comes again to rob you you will be ready; you still trust him. So the person who was deceiving you may have robbed you materially, but he has enriched you spiritually.

But what happens ordinarily? One man deceives you and the whole humanity is condemned. One Christian deceives you; all Christians are condemned. One Mohammedan has not behaved well with you; the whole community of Mohammedans are sinners. One Hindu has not been good to you; all Hindus are worthless. You simply wait. Just a single man can create a distrust of the whole humanity.

A man of trust goes on trusting. Whatsoever happens to his trust, one thing never happens: he never allows anybody to destroy his trust. His trust goes on increasing. Trust is God. People have told you to trust in God; I tell you, trust *is* God. Forget all about God; just trust, and God will come seeking and searching for you wherever you are.

The second question:

What motivates a Buddha?

The question is absurd, because a Buddha becomes a Buddha only when all motivation has left, when all desires have disappeared. A Buddha becomes a Buddha only because he now has nothing to do, nothing to desire, nowhere to go, no achievement. The achieving mind disappears—then one becomes a Buddha. So if you ask, "What motivates a Buddha?" you are asking an absurd question. Nothing can motivate him; that's why he is a Buddha.

Siddhartha Gautama became enlightened. The story goes that a Brahmin was passing by. He had never seen such a beautiful person. Something unearthly was surrounding Buddha sitting under his tree; he was luminous, a tremendous peace. The Brahmin could not go. He was in a hurry, he had to reach somewhere; but the silence of Buddha pulled him. He forgot where he was going, he forgot his motivation. Being close to this man who had attained to the state of no motivation, he was pulled into his whirlpool. Enchanted, he remained there, the story says, for hours. Then suddenly he became aware; what was he doing there? Then he suddenly became aware that he was going somewhere, but where? Then he asked, "Who am I"—as if the whole identity, the whole past had somewhere disappeared. He could not bring who he was to his consciousness. Then he shook Buddha and he said, "What have you done to me? I have completely forgotten where I was going, and from where I was coming, and who I am. Now who am I going to ask? Who will answer this? And I am a stranger to this part of the country. You tell me what you have done!" Buddha opened his eyes and he said, "I have not done anything. I have stopped doing. Maybe because of it, maybe just being close to me . . . you don't be worried. You run away from me fast." The man said, "Before I go, one thing I have to ask: are you a God?" He had heard, he was a learned Brahmin. He had recited the Vedas every day as part of ritual, daily ritual. He had heard about Krishna and Ram, but they had remained just stories. For the first time somebody seemed to be there—solid, real, earthly, and still divine: "Are you a God?" Buddha said, "No." The man said, "Are you a saint, an *arhat?*"—because the man understood. In India Jains don't believe in God, so when somebody attains to the perfect, ultimate truth, he is called an arhat: one who has arrived; the sage, the saint. So first he asked, "Are you a God?" He asked a question in the terminology of the Hindus, and Buddha said, "No." Then he thought, "Maybe he belongs to the other tradition of the Indians, the tradition of the *shramanas* who don't believe in God." He asked, "Are you an arhat, a sage, a saint?" and Buddha said, "No." Then he was puzzled because these were the only two languages possible. Then he said, "Then who are you?" Buddha said, "I am aware." It is not very grammatical, but true. He said, "I am aware." He simply indicated the quality of his being at that moment—awareness—not God, not saint. Because when you say 'God', it seems something is static. When you say 'saint', it seems something is complete, static, has become a thing. Buddha said, "I am aware." Or, an even better translation: he said, "I am awareness"—no identity, just a dynamic energy of being aware. In awareness, in such awareness there is no motivation; and if there is motivation, there is no awareness.

Let me tell you one anecdote, a very beautiful one. Listen to it as deeply as possible.

The lady and her small son were swimming in the surf, and there was a very heavy undertow. She was holding her son tightly by the hand and they were splashing around happily, when a huge wall of water loomed up ahead of them. As they watched in horror, this tidal wave rose higher and higher directly in front of them, and crashed over them. When the water receded, the little boy was nowhere to be found. Panic-stricken, the mother searched in the water screaming, "Melvyn, Melvyn, where are you? Melvyn!" When it was obvious the child was lost, washed out to the sea, the distraught mother lifted her eyes to heaven and prayed, "Oh, dear and merciful Father, please take pity on me and return my beautiful child. I will promise eternal gratitude to you. I promise I will never cheat on my husband again; I will never cheat on my income tax again; I will be kind to my mother-in-law; I will give up smoking; anything! Anything, only please grant me this one favor and return my son."

Just then, another wall of water loomed up and crashed over her head. When the water receded, there was her small son standing there. She clasped him to her bosom, kissed him, clung to him. Then she looked at him a moment, and once again turned her eyes heavenward. Looking up, she said, "But he had a hat."

This is the mind: the son is back but the hat is lost. Now she was not happy because the son was back, but unhappy because the hat was lost—again complaining.

Have you watched this happening inside your mind, or not? It is always happening. Whatsoever life gives to you, you are not thankful for it. You are again and again complaining about the hat. You always go on seeing that which has not happened, not that which has already happened. You always look and desire and expect, but you are never grateful. Millions of things are happening to you, but you are never grateful. You always remain grumpy, complaining, and you are always in a state of frustration. Even if you reach to heaven, this mind will not allow you to live there. You will create a hell wherever you are: so much desire that one desire is fulfilled, ten desires arise out of it; and it never comes to an end.

By desiring, no one has ever attained to the state of peace, the state of non-desire. By understanding the desire, by understanding the motivation, one becomes, by and by, alert. One comes to know that if you drop motivation, there is no frustration in life. Then nothing can make you unhappy. Then happiness is natural; it is just the way you are. Then whatsoever happens, you remain happy. Now, whatsoever happens, you remain unhappy.

A Buddha has no motivation; that's why he's happy. He's so happy that if you ask him, "Are you happy?" he will shrug his shoulders—because how to know? Happiness can be known only in contrast to unhappiness. He has forgotten the very experience of unhappiness, so if you ask him, "Are you happy?" he may keep quiet. He may not say anything. Because when unhappiness disappeared, with it disappeared that dichotomy also. That's why Buddha has not said that the ultimate state is that of bliss. No, he says it is of peace, but not of bliss.

That is one of the differences between Hindus and Buddhists, between Patanjali and Buddha. That is one of the basic differences. And of course, both are right; these things are such when you talk about the ultimate, if you know about it. So whatsoever you say, howsoever contradictory it appears, it is always right. Patanjali says that it is a state of bliss because all misery, all possibility of misery has disappeared. Of course, he is right. Buddha says, "It is not even bliss, because who will know and how will you know that it is blissful? When all misery has disappeared, there is no contrast, there is no way to know it." If nights disappear completely, how will you know that this is day? It will be day, but how will you know it is day? Buddha is also right: it will be bliss, but it cannot be called bliss because to say so, you bring unhappiness in.

One becomes a Buddha when one has understood the mechanism of all motivation. What is motivation?—it is a discontent in the present, an uneasiness in the present, and a hope in the future. Motivation is a discontent here-now, and a dream of contentment somewhere in the future.

You live in a small house: you are unhappy with this small house, discontented here-now, and you hope for a bigger house in the future. Future is needed; right now the big house is not possible. Time will be needed to make, to earn money, to do a thousand and one things, to compete. Then, the big house will be possible. So right now you are in discontent, but in future you have a dream of contentment. You work hard. Then the big house becomes possible one day, but suddenly you see nothing like contentment is happening to you. The moment the big house becomes available, you start thinking of bigger houses. You have become addicted to motivation. Now you cannot live without motivation. Again in the big house, you are unhappy. Again you are hoping: "Someday, some palace, somewhere"—and this is how one goes on wasting one's whole life.

Understand the mechanism of motivation. It gives you a dream in the future—and a dream is a dream—and it takes all blissfulness from the present. For something unreal, it destroys that which is real. Once you understand, you stop living through motivation. Then you live simply without motivation.

What is without, what is living without motivation?—living in deep contentment here and now, and not bothering for the tomorrow.

Says Jesus, "Think not of the morrow. Look at the lillies of the field. Even King Solomon was not so beautiful in all his grandeur. Look at the lilies in the field; they don't think of the morrow. They are just here and now. They are with God here and now. They don't have any future; they don't carry the past. This moment is all."

A mind which has dropped motivation is no more a mind. Once you drop motivation, you have become part of the eternal reality which is always now, always here. And then you are contented. Out of your contentment, more contentment arises; bigger and bigger waves of contentment arise. Out of your discontent, more and more discontent arises.

So look . . . this moment you can move into the world of motivation in which you are already moving—the competition, the market-place—or, you can move in the world of non-motivation. At each step the paths bifurcate. If you drop motivation, you decide to be happy right this moment and you say, "Let the future take its own care. Now I will be here and now, and that's all, and I don't ask more. I will enjoy that which is already given to me." And more than enough is given to you already.

I have never seen a man who is not rich in life, but it is very difficult to find a rich man—all are beggars. And I tell you, nobody need be a beggar. Life has given so many riches to you already, that if you know how to enjoy them you will not ask more. You will say, "Even this much I cannot enjoy. This is too much already. I cannot hold it. My hands are too small, my heart is so small; I cannot hold it! You have given me so much dance, and so much song, and so much blissfulness. More I cannot ask. Even to exhaust this is not possible."

To live here-now is to be religious. To live here-now is to live without mind. To live here-now is to become a Buddha. That's what he said: "I am aware." Because Gods are also motivated, they are also chasing women—maybe better women on some higher plane, but chasing women. They are competitive with each other.

Hindus are tremendously beautiful about this. They have not shrunk back about anything. If you listen to God's stories in Hindu *Puranas*, you will be tremendously surprised: they are almost human. They are doing all the same things that you are doing—maybe in a little better way, or maybe on a little higher plane. The head, the chief God is called Indra. He is the King of Gods. And he is always afraid—as kings always are—and his throne is always shaking because somebody is always pulling his legs. You can go to Delhi and ask people. Whenever you are on a throne somebody is pulling, many are pulling in fact, because they also want to be on the throne. Indra is continuously trembling. I think, by now, trembling must have become a habit to him. Whether anybody is pulling or not, he must be trembling. For centuries he has been trembling. Stories say that whenever some ascetic, some saint on the earth starts achieving higher planes of being, he starts feeling afraid. His throne starts shaking; somebody is trying to be competitive with him. Somebody is trying to become a king of Gods. Immediately he sends beautiful damsels, *apsaras*, to destroy that poor ascetic. They dance a beautiful, sexual dance around him; they seduce the poor ascetic. And then Indra sleeps well: now one competitor is destroyed.

In the Hindu heaven the paths are studded with diamonds, and the trees are of gold, and flowers are of silver and jade and jewels—but the same world. Women are very beautiful there—but the same world, the same lust, the same desire. Hindus say, "Even Gods will have to be reborn on earth when their virtue is finished, when they have enjoyed their *punya*, their virtue."

This word 'punya' is very good. 'Poona' comes out of *punya*. It means: the city of virtue. Those Gods are as worldly as this world.

They will have to come back once their punya, their virtue, is finished. Once they have enjoyed then they have to come back to the earth, to crawl again.

Buddha says, "No, I am not a God, because I have no motivation." "Are you a saint, an *arhata?*" Buddha says, "No, because even a saint has a certain motivation to achieve liberation"—how to achieve *moksha*, how to go beyond the world, how to become desireless. But still, the desire is there. Now the desire is of becoming desireless. Motivation can be of becoming motiveless: how to achieve a state of non-motivation—that can become a motivation. But it is all the same; you are again in the same trap.

Buddha says, "No, I am aware." In awareness, motivation does not arise. So whenever motivation arises, a desire arises. Don't do anything. Just be aware, and you will see the desire is receding back, disappearing. It evaporates. When the sun of awareness arises, desires evaporate like dew-drops in the morning.

The third question:

If enlightened beings don't have children, and we neurotic people are pronounced unfit for parenthood by you, when is the right time?

Enlightened persons don't have children; neurotic persons should not have. Just between the two, there is a state of mental health, of non-neurosis: you are neither neurotic nor enlightened, simply healthy. Just in the middle—that is the right time for parenthood, to become a mother or to become a father.

This is the trouble: neurotic persons tend to have many children. In fact, in the West neurosis is more. People don't have many children. That may be one of the causes that neurosis has become so prevalent: the old engagement with children is no longer there. In the East, people are not so neurotic. They cannot afford to be neurotic; children are enough. A joint family has so many children. You cannot have any time to go mad—impossible. They won't allow you to. You are in such a mad state and so tuned with it, that you will not become aware that you are mad. In the West, the joint family has disappeared. Children have also disappeared, the way they appear in the East. There are one or two children, at the most.

Much space is left. The whole old occupation is no longer there. People are becoming more and more rich, affluent, less and less work is there, more and more leisure, and they don't know what to do with the leisure. They go neurotic. Just think about yourself if you have nothing to do, no children to work for.

Once I asked Mulla Nasrudin, "Are you still working for the same firm?" He said, "Yes, the same company: the wife and thirteen kids!"

If you have a family to support, to work hard for the whole life, from morning till evening, and you come home tired and go to sleep and in the morning you are again on the track, how can you afford to be neurotic? When will you find time to go to a psychiatrist? In the East the psychiatrist does not exist. Children are the only psychiatrists.

Neurotic persons tend, in their neurosis, to create a very occupied space around them. They should not, because that is avoiding. They should face the fact of neurosis and they should go beyond it.

An enlightened person need not have children. He has given the ultimate birth to himself. Now there is no need to give birth to anything else. He has become a father and mother to himself. He has become a womb to himself, and he is reborn.

But between the two, when the neurosis is not there, you meditate, you become a little alert, aware. Your life is not just of darkness. The light is not as penetrating as it is when one becomes a Buddha, but a dim candlelight is available. That is the right time—the twilight time, when you are just on the border, moving out of the world, moving in the other world; that is the right time to have children, because then you will be able to give something of your awareness to your children. Otherwise, what will you give as a gift to them? You will give your neurosis.

I have heard: A man with eighteen children took them to a dairy show. Included in the show was a prize bull worth 8,000 pounds and there was an additional charge of five pence to go in and see it. The man thought that this charge was exorbitant, but his children wanted to see the animal, and so they approached the entrance to its enclosure. The attendant said, "Are all these children yours, sir?"

"Yes, they are," answered the man. "Why?"

The attendant replied, "Well, wait here a minute and I will bring the bull out to see you!"

Eighteen children!—even the bull will feel jealous.

You go on unconsciously reproducing your own replicas. First think: are you in such a state that if you give birth to a child, you will be giving a gift to the world? Are you a blessing to the world, or a curse? And then think: are you ready to mother or to father a child? Are you ready to give love unconditionally? Because children come through you, but they don't belong to you. You can give your love to them, but you should not impose your ideas on them. You should not give your neurotic styles to them. Are you ready not to give your neurotic style to your children? Will you allow them to flower in their own way? Will you allow them freedom to be themselves? If you are ready, then it is okay. Otherwise, wait; become ready.

With man, conscious evolution has entered into the world. Don't be like animals, just reproducing unconsciously. Now get ready before you would like to have a child. Become more meditative, become more quiet and peaceful. Get rid of all the neurosis that you have within you. Wait for that moment when you are absolutely clean, then give birth to a child. Then, give your life to the child, your love to the child. You will be helping to create a better world. Otherwise, you will be simply crowding the world. The crowd has already become maddening. There is no longer any need to increase the crowd. If you can give human beings to the world, not just like worms, crowding and crawling all over the earth, then first be ready.

To me, to become a mother is a great discipline; to become a father is a great austerity. Otherwise, you will leave somebody just like you, or even worse than you, in your place. That will not be a good gesture on your part. Enlightened people need not give birth to anybody; neurotic people should not. Just in between the two, is the point.

The last question:

You say, remove all your masks and be authentic. I think only of
sex, love and romance. I don't know anything else except this.
Am I on the wrong track?

I don't see anything wrong in sex, in love, in romance. You are on the right track. Love is the right track, and only through a lived life of love, prayer arises—never otherwise. Only out of deep experiences of love, sweet and bitter, pleasant and painful, high and low, heaven and hell; only out of deep experiences of pain and pleasure through love does one become aware. They are needed to make you aware.

Pain is as much needed as pleasure, because both work. And by and by, between the pleasure and the pain, you become a tightrope walker. You attain to balance.

But for centuries love has been condemned, sex has been condemned. So of course, the idea arises in your mind that you must be on the wrong track. You are simply natural. To be natural is not to be the wrong track. If you think in that way and you become condemnatory, then you will be on the wrong track. Then you will repress, and whatsoever you repress will remain lurking in your unconscious, in your basement, and then much ugliness arises out of that repression.

Let me tell you a few anecdotes.

It is said about a very rich and well known man, Lord Dewsberry: he was ninety years old to the day, and sat in the large bay window of his ground floor flat in Park Lane watching the Sunday morning strollers. Suddenly, he spotted a pretty, young, and fair girl wheeling a pram across to the park. "Quickly James," he said. "My teeth; I want to whistle."

Ninety years old!—but this happens.

The question is from Krishna Priya.

Remember, if you don't whistle now, then someday when your teeth are also gone, you will see some young man walking and, "Quick, bring my teeth!" That will be ugly. Right now the teeth are okay; you can whistle. Everything should be done in its time. Otherwise, things become ugly.

A child running after butterflies is okay, but a man of forty running around butterflies will look mad. Young men are bound to be a little foolish. One expects that and accepts also. Nothing is wrong in it. That must be something basic to life: to be foolish at some times, because wisdom comes out of the experience of many foolishnesses. You cannot become wise suddenly. You will have to move, and go astray, and do many foolish things. And out of all those actions, foolish or otherwise, wisdom arises.

Wisdom is like fragrance, and experiences of foolishness work like manure. They stink!—but beautiful flowers come out of them. So don't avoid the manure of life, otherwise you will miss the flowers of wisdom. And you can repress one desire from one side, but it will start arising from another side. You cannot deceive life.

"Mummy," said the little monster, "the lads at school keep saying I have got a very big head."

"You have not got a big head at all," said the mother. "Just forget about those nasty boys and pop down to the shops for me. I want ten pounds of potatoes, five pounds of turnips, and two cabbages."

"Alright, mummy. Where is the shopping bag?"

"Oh, don't bother about that. Just use your cap."

So from this way or that . . . just think again. Ten pounds of potatoes, five pounds of turnips and two cabbages—and just use your hat, just use your cap. You can suppress from one side; it bubbles up from another side. Never suppress anything. If sex is there, allow it before it is too late. Allow it, move into it, accept it. It is a God-given thing. There must be a deep reason in it. There is. Never shirk any responsibility that God has given to you, otherwise you shirk from growth. And now, to ask such questions in this century, this twentieth century, is simply stupid.

The six-year-old was having his first trip to the zoo, and was asking awkward questions as usual. "Hey Dad, where do baby elephants come from?" he asked; then added, "and if you give me that old stork story this time, I will really know you are crazy."

Elephants being brought by the stork?—so the six-year-old is saying, "And if you give me that old stork story this time, I will really know you are crazy."

Gone are those foolish days when people were thinking in terms of condemnation, of anti-life philosophies. After Freud, man has come to accept sex more naturally. A great revolution has happened in the world.

Now to think in condemnatory ways is simply not to be contemporary. Now, Krishna Priya's question was okay if she had asked it five hundred years ago, but now? It is absurd.

And in my ashram?

CHAPTER NINE
May 9, 1976

KAIVALYA

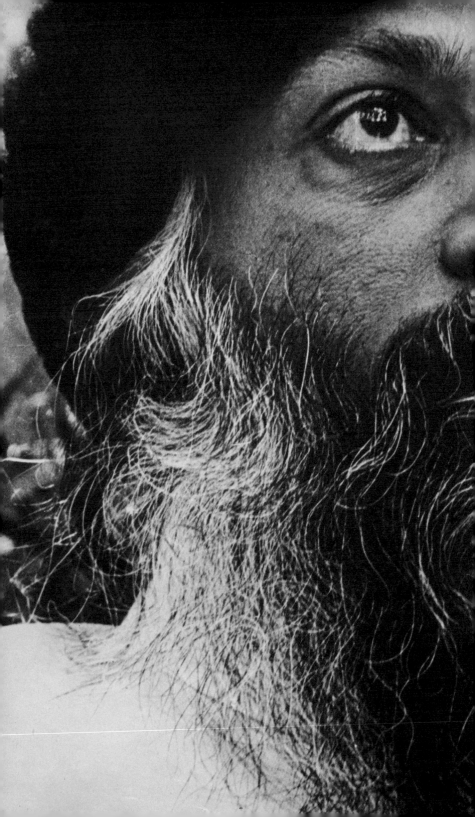

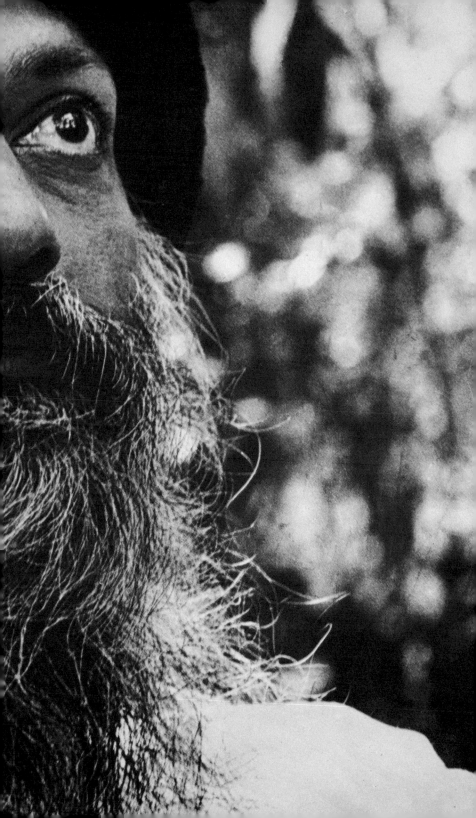

25

When one has seen this distinction, there is a cessation of desire for dwelling in the atma, the self.

विशेषदर्शिन आत्मभावभावनाविनिवृत्तिः ॥ २५ ॥

26

Then the mind is inclined towards discrimination, and gravitates towards liberation.

तदा विवेकनिम्नं कैवल्यप्राग्भारं चित्तम् ॥ २६ ॥

27

In breaks of discrimination, other pratyayas, concepts, arise through the force of previous impressions. These should be removed in the same way as other afflictions.

तच्छिद्रेषु प्रत्ययान्तराणि संस्कारेभ्यः ॥ २७ ॥

28

One who is able to maintain a constant state of desirelessness even towards the most exalted states of enlightenment, and is able to exercise the highest kind of discrimination, enters the state known as 'the cloud which showers virtue'.

हानमेषां क्लेशवदुक्तम् ॥ २८ ॥

29

Then follows freedom from afflictions and karmas.

प्रसंख्यानेऽप्यकुसीदस्य सर्वथा विवेकख्यातेर्धर्ममेघः समाधिः ॥ २९ ॥

30

That which can be known through the mind is very little compared with the infinite knowledge obtained in enlightenment, when the veils, distortions, and impurities are removed.

ततः क्लेशकर्मनिवृत्तिः ॥ ३० ॥

31

Having fulfilled their object, the process of change in the three gunas comes to an end.

तदा सर्वावरणमलापेतस्य ज्ञानस्यानन्त्याज्ज्ञेयमल्पम् ॥ ३१ ॥

32

Kramaha, the process, is the succession of changes that occur from moment to moment which become apprehensible at the final end of the transformations of the three gunas.

ततः कृतार्थानां परिणामक्रमसमाप्तिर्गुणानाम् ॥ ३२ ॥

33

Kaivalya is the state of enlightenment that follows the remergence of the gunas, due to their becoming devoid of the object of the Purusa.

क्षणप्रतियोगी परिणामापरान्तनिर्ब्राह्यः क्रमः ॥ ३३ ॥

34

In this state, the Purusa is established in his real nature, which is pure consciousness.

पुरुषार्थशून्यानां गुणानां प्रति प्रसवः कैवल्यं स्वरूपप्रतिष्ठा वा

The first sutra:

Visesa-darsina atma-bhava-bhavanavinivṛttih.

*When one has seen this distinction, there is a
cessation of desire for dwelling in the atma, the self.*

BUDDHA HAS CALLED THE ULTIMATE STATE OF CON-
SCIOUSNESS *ANATTA*—NO SELF, NON-BEING. It is
very difficult to comprehend it. Buddha has said that the
last desire to drop is the desire to be. There are millions of
desires. The whole world is nothing but desire objects, but the basic
desire is to be. The basic desire is to continue, to persist, to remain.
Death is the greatest fear; the last desire to be dropped is the desire
to be.

Patanjali in this sutra says: when your awareness has become
perfect, when *viveka*, discrimination has been achieved, when you
have become a witness, a pure witness of whatsoever happens,
outside you, inside you. . . . You are no more a doer, you are simply
watching; the birds are singing outside . . . you watch; the blood is
circulating inside . . . you watch; the thoughts are moving inside . . .
you watch—you never get identified anywhere. You don't say, "I
am the body"; you don't say, "I am the mind"; you don't say
anything. You simply go on watching without being identified with
any object. You remain a pure subject; you simply remember one
thing: that you are the watcher, the witness—when this witnessing
is established, then the desire to be disappears.

And the moment the desire to be disappears, death also disappears. Death exists because you want to persist. Death exists because you don't want to die. Death exists because you are struggling against the whole. The moment you are ready to die, death
is meaningless; it cannot be possible now. When you are ready to
die, how can you die? In the very readiness of dying, disappearing,
all possibility of death is overcome. This is the paradox of religion.

Jesus says, "If you are going to cling to yourself, you will lose
yourself. If you want to attain yourself, don't cling." Those who try
to be are destroyed. Not that somebody is there destroying you;
your very effort to be is destructive because the moment the idea
arises: "I should persist," you are moving against the whole. It is as

if a wave is trying to be against the ocean. Now the very effort is going to create worry and misery, and one moment will come when the wave will have to disappear. But now, because the wave was fighting against the ocean, the disappearance will look like death. If the wave was ready, and the wave was aware: "I'm nothing but the ocean, so what is the point in persisting? I have been always and I will be always, because the ocean has always been there and will be always there. I may not exist as a wave—wave is just the form I have taken for the moment. The form will disappear, but not my content. I may not exist like *this* wave; I may exist like another wave, or I may not exist as a wave as such. I may become the very depth of the ocean where no waves arise. . . ."

But the innermost reality is going to remain because the whole has penetrated you. You are nothing but the whole, an expression of the whole. Once awareness is established, Patanjali says, "When one has seen this distinction, that 'I am neither this nor that', when one has become aware and is not identified with anything whatsoever, there is a cessation of desire for dwelling in the *atma*, in the self." Then the last desire disappears, and the last is the fundamental. Hence, Buddha says, "You can drop desiring money, wealth, power, prestige—that's nothing. You can stop desiring the world—that's nothing—because those are secondary desires. The basic desire is to be." So people who renounce the world start desiring liberation, but liberation is also *their* liberation. They will remain in *moksha*, in a liberated state. They desire that pain should not be there. They desire that misery should not be there. They will be in absolute bliss, but they will be. The insistence is that they must be there.

That's why Buddha could not get roots into this country which thinks itself very religious. The most religious man who was born on this earth could not get roots into this religious country. What happened? He said, he insisted, to drop the basic desire of being: he said, "Be a non-being." He said, "Don't be." He said, "Don't ask for liberation because the freedom is not for you. The freedom is going to be freedom from you; not for you, but from you."

Liberation is liberation from yourself. See the distinction: it is not for you; liberation is not for you. It is not that liberated you will exist. Liberated, you will disappear. Buddha said, "Only bondage exists." Let me try to explain it to you.

Have you ever come across health? You have been healthy many times, but can you say what health is? Only disease exists. Health is non-existential; you cannot pin-point it. If you have a headache you know it is there, but have you ever known the absence of headache? In fact, if there is no headache the head also disappears. You don't feel it anymore. If you go on feeling your head, that simply shows that there must be a certain tension inside, a certain stress, a strain. A sort of headache must be there continuously. If your whole body is healthy, the body disappears. You forget that the body is. In Zen, when meditators sit for many years, just sitting and doing nothing, a certain moment comes when they forget that they have bodies. That is their first *satori*. Not that the body is not there; body is there but there is no tension, so how to feel it? If I say something you can hear me, but if I'm silent how can you hear me? Silence is there—it has much to communicate to you—but silence cannot be heard. Sometimes when you say, "Yes, I can hear the silence," then you are hearing some noise. Maybe it is the noise of the dark night, but it is still noise. If it is absolutely silent, you will not be able to hear it. When your body is perfectly healthy, you don't feel it. If some tension arises in the body, some disease, some illness, then you start hearing. If everything is in harmony and there is no pain and no misery, suddenly you are empty. A nothingness overwhelms you.

Kaivalya is the ultimate health, wholeness, all wounds healed. When all wounds heal, how can you exist? The self is nothing but accumulated tensions. The self is nothing but all sorts of diseases, illnesses. The self is nothing but desires unfulfilled, hopes frustrated, expectations, dreams—all broken, fractured. It is nothing but accumulated disease, that you call 'self'. Or take it from another side: in moments of harmony you forget that you are. Later on, you may remember how beautiful it was, how fantastic it was, how far-out. But in moments of real far-outness, you are not there. Something bigger than you has overpowered you; something higher than you has possessed you; something deeper than you has bubbled up. You have disappeared. In deep moments of love, lovers disappear. In deep moments of silence, meditators disappear. In deep moments of singing, dancing, celebration, celebrators disappear. And this is going to be the last celebration, the ultimate, the highest peak—*kaivalya*.

Patanjali says, "Even the desire to be disappears. Even the desire to remain disappears." One is so fulfilled, so tremendously fulfilled that one never thinks in terms of being. For what?—you want to be there tomorrow also because today is unfulfilled. The tomorrow is needed; otherwise you will die unfulfilled. The yesterday was a deep frustration; today is again a frustration; tomorrow is needed.

A frustrated mind creates future. A frustrated mind clings with the future. A frustrated mind wants to be because now, if death comes, no flower has flowered. Nothing has yet happened; there has only been a fruitless waiting: "Now, how can I die? I have not even lived yet." That unlived life creates a desire to be.

People are so much afraid of death: these are the people who have not lived. These are the people who are, in a certain sense, already dead. A person who has lived and lived totally does not think about death. If it comes, good; he will welcome. He will live that too, he will celebrate that too. Life has been such a blessing, a benediction; one is even ready to accept death. Life has been such a tremendous experience; one is ready to experience death also. One is not afraid because the tomorrow is not needed; the today has been so fulfilling. One has come to fruition, flowered, bloomed. Now the desire for tomorrow disappears. The desire for tomorrow is always out of fear, and fear is there because love has not happened. The desire to always remain simply shows that deep down you are feeling yourself completely meaningless. You are waiting for some meaning. Once the meaning has happened, you are ready to die—silently, beautifully, gracefully.

"Kaivalya," Patanjali says, "happens only when the last desire to be has disappeared." The whole problem is to be or not to be. The whole life we try to be this and that, and the ultimate can happen only when you are not.

When one has seen this distinction, there is a
cessation of desire for dwelling in the self.

The self is nothing but the most purified form of the ego. It is the last remnant of strain, stress, tension. You are still not perfectly open; something is still closed. When you are completely open, just a watcher on the hill, a witness, even the death desire disappears. With the disappearance of this desire, something absolutely new happens in life. A new law starts functioning.

You have heard about the law of gravitation; you have not heard about the law of grace. The law of gravitation is that everything falls downwards. The law of grace is that things start falling upwards. And that law has to be there because in life everything is balanced by the opposite. Science has come to discover the law of gravitation: Newton sitting on a bench in a garden saw one apple falling—it happened or not; that is not the point—but seeing that the apple was falling down, a thought arose in him: "Why do things always fall downwards? Why not otherwise? Why doesn't a ripe fruit fall upwards and disappear into the sky? Why not sideways? Why always downwards?" He started brooding and meditating, and then he discovered a law. He came upon, stumbled upon a very fundamental law: that the earth is gravitating things towards itself. It has a gravitation field. Like a magnet, it pulls everything downwards.

Patanjali, Buddha, Krishna, Christ—they also became aware of a different fundamental law, higher than gravitation. They became aware that there comes a moment in the inner life of consciousness when consciousness starts rising upwards—exactly like gravitation. If the apple is hanging on the tree, it does not fall. The tree helps it not to fall downwards. When the fruit leaves the tree, then it falls downwards.

Exactly the same: if you are clinging to your body you will not fall upwards; if you are clinging to your mind you will not fall upwards. If you are clinging to the idea of self, you will remain under the impact of gravitation—because body is under the impact of gravitation, and mind also. Mind is subtle body; body is gross mind. They are both under the impact of gravitation. And because you are clinging to them you are not under the impact of gravitation, but you are clinging to something which is under the impact of gravitation. It is as if you are carrying a big rock and trying to swim in a river; the rock will pull you down. It won't allow you to swim. If you leave the rock, you will be able to swim easily.

We are clinging to something which is functioning under the law of gravitation: body, mind. "Once," Patanjali says, "you have become aware that you are neither the body nor the mind, suddenly you start rising upwards." Some center somewhere high in the sky pulls you up. That law is called 'grace'. Then God pulls you upwards. And that type of law has to be there, otherwise gravitation could not exist. In nature, if positive electricity exists, then negative electricity has to exist. Man exists, then the woman has to exist. Reason exists, then intuition has to exist. Night exists, then the day has to exist. Life exists, then death has to exist. Everything needs the opposite to balance it. Now science has become aware of one law: gravitation. Science still needs a Patanjali to give it another dimension, the dimension of falling upwards. Then life becomes complete.

You are a meeting place of gravitation and grace. In you, grace and gravitation are criss-crossing. You have something of the earth and something of the sky within you. You are the horizon where earth and sky are meeting. If you hold too much to the earth, then you will forget completely that you belong to the sky, to the infinite space, the beyond. Once you are no more attached with the earth part of you, suddenly you start rising high.

> *When one has seen this distinction, there is a*
> *cessation of desire for dwelling in the self.*
>
> *Tadahi viveka-nimnam kaivalya-pragbharam cittam.*
>
> *Then the mind is inclined towards discrimination,*
> *and gravitates towards liberation.*

A new gravitation starts functioning. Liberation is nothing but entering the stream of grace. You cannot liberate yourself, you can only drop the barriers; liberation happens to you. Have you seen a magnet?—small iron pieces are pulled towards it. You can see those small iron pieces rushing towards the magnet, but don't be deceived by your eyes. In fact, they are not rushing, the magnet is pulling them. On the surface it appears that those iron filings are going, moving towards the magnet. That is just on the surface. Deep down, something just opposite is happening: they are not moving towards the magnet, the magnet is pulling them towards itself. In fact, it is the magnet which has reached them. With the magnetic field it has approached them, touched them, pulled them. If those iron filings are free, not attached to something—not attached to a rock—then the magnet can pull them. If they are attached to a rock, the magnet will go on pulling but they will not be pulled because they are attached.

Exactly the same happens: once you discriminate that you are not the body, you are no more bound to any rock, you are no more in bondage with earth. Immediately, God's magnet starts functioning. It is not that you reach to God. In fact, God has already reached you. You are under His magnetic field, but clinging to something. Drop that clinging and you are in the stream. Buddha used to use a word *srotaapanna:* falling into the stream. He used to say, "Once you fall into the stream, then the stream takes you to the ocean. Then you need not do anything." The only thing is to jump into the stream. You are sitting on the bank. Enter the stream and then the stream will do the remaining work. It is as if you are standing on a high building, on the roof of a high building, three hundred feet or five hundred feet above the earth. You go on standing, the gravitation has reached you, but it will not work unless you jump. Once you jump, then you need not do anything. Just a step off the roof . . . enough; your work is finished. Now the gravitation will do all the work. You need not ask, "Now what am I supposed to do?" You have taken the first step. The first is the last step. Krishnamurti has written a book, *The First and the Last Freedom*. The meaning is: the first step is the last step—because once you are in the stream, everything else is to be done by the stream. You are not needed. Only for the first step is your courage needed.

> *Then the mind is inclined towards discrimination,*
> *and gravitates towards liberation.*

You start moving slowly upwards. Your life energy starts rising high—an upsurge. And it is unbelievable when it happens because it is against all the laws that you have known up to now. It is levitation, not gravitation. Something in you simply starts moving upwards, and there is no barrier to it. Nothing bars its path. Just a little relaxation, a little unclinging—the first step—and then automatically, spontaneously, your consciousness becomes more and more discriminative, more and more aware.

Let me tell you about another thing. You have heard the word, the phrase: 'vicious circle'. Let us make another phrase: 'virtuous circle'. In a vicious circle, one bad thing leads to another. For example, if you get angry then one anger leads you to more anger, and of course, more anger will lead you to still more anger. Now you are in a vicious circle. Each anger will make the habit of anger more strong, and will create more anger, and more anger will make the habit still more strong, and on and on. You move in a vicious circle which goes on becoming stronger and stronger and stronger.

Let us try a new word: virtuous circle. If you become aware, what Patanjali calls *vivek*, awareness; if you become aware: *vairagya*. Discrimination creates renunciation. If you become aware, suddenly you see that you are no more the body. Not that you renounce the body; in your very awareness the body is renounced. If you become aware, you become aware that these thoughts are not you. In that very awareness those thoughts are renounced. You have started dropping them. You don't give them any more energy; you don't cooperate with them. Your cooperation has stopped, and they cannot live without your energy. They live on your energy, they exploit you. They don't have their own energy. Each thought that enters you partakes of your energy. And because you are willing to give your energy, it lives there, it makes its abode there. Of course, then its children come, and friends, and relatives, and this goes on. Once you are a little aware, *vivek* brings *vairagya*, awareness brings renunciation. And renunciation makes you capable of becoming more aware. And of course, more awareness brings more *vairagya*, more renunciation, and so on and so forth.

This is what I am calling the virtuous circle: one virtue leads to another, and each virtue becomes again a ground for more virtue to arise.

"This goes on," Patanjali says, "to the last moment"—what he calls, *dharma megha samadhi*. We will be coming to it later on. He calls it 'the cloud of virtue showering on you'. This virtuous circle, *vivek* leading to *vairagya*, *vairagya* leading to more *vivek*, *vivek* again creating more possibilities for *vairagya*, and so on and so forth— comes to the ultimate peak when the cloud of virtue showers on you: *dharma megha samadhi*.

> *In breaks of discrimination, other pratyayas,*
> *concepts, arise through the force of previous*
> *impressions.*

Still, though, many intervals will be there. So don't be discouraged. Even if you have become very aware and in sudden moments you feel the pull, the upward pull of grace, and in certain moments you are in the stream, floating perfectly beautifully, with no effort, effortlessly, and everything is going and running smoothly, still there will be gaps. Suddenly you will find yourself standing again on the bank just because of old habits. For so many lives you have lived on the bank. Just because of the old habit, again and again the past will overpower you. Don't be discouraged by it. The moment you see that you are again on the bank, again get down into the stream. Don't be sad about it, because if you become sad you will again be in a vicious circle. Don't be sad about it. Many times the seeker comes at very close quarters, and many times he loses the track. No need to be worried; again bring awareness. This is going to happen many times; it is natural. For so many millions of lives we have lived in unawareness—it is only natural that many times the old habit will start functioning. Let me tell you a few anecdotes.

The boss was full of confidence as he approached the reception desk at a large hotel with his secretary and signed the register as Mr. and Mrs.

"Double or twin beds?" enquired the clerk.

He turned to his secretary and asked casually, "Would a double be alright, darling?"

"Yes, sir," she answered.

"Yes, sir," the wife was saying to the husband!—but just the old habit of being a secretary, continuously saying, "Yes sir, yes sir, yes sir." Habits become very ingrained, and they catch hold of you in such a way that unless you are very, very watchful, you will not even suspect.

It happened: An indignant schoolteacher rang the local police station to complain that a crowd of young hooligans had chalked four-letter words all over her front door. "And what is more," she concluded, "they have not even spelled them right!"

A school teacher is just a school teacher. She is complaining against the four-letter words, but the basic complaint is that they have not even spelled them right. Continuously correcting the spelling of children. . . .

> In breaks of discrimination, other concepts arise
> through the force of previous impressions.

Many times you will be pulled back, again and again and again. The struggle is hard, but not impossible. It is difficult, it is very arduous, but don't become sad and don't become discouraged. Whenever you remember again, don't be worried about what has happened. Let your awareness again be established, that's all. Continuously establishing your awareness again and again and again will create a new impact inside your being, a new impression of virtue. One day, it becomes as natural as other habits.

> One who is able to maintain a constant state of
> desirelessness, even towards the most exalted states
> of enlightenment, and is able to exercise the highest
> kind of discrimination, enters the state known as 'the
> cloud which showers virtue'.

"One who is able to maintain a constant state of desirelessness even towards the most exalted states of enlightenment . . ." Patanjali calls it *paravairagya*: the ultimate renunciation. You have renounced the world: you have renounced greed, you have renounced money, you have renounced power; you have renounced everything of the outside. You have even renounced your body, you have even renounced your mind, but the last renunciation is the renunciation of *kaivalya* itself, of *moksha* itself, of *nirvana* itself. Now you renounce even the idea of liberation, because that too is a desire. And desire, whatsoever its object, is the same. You desire money, I desire moksha. Of course, my object is better than your object, but still my desire is the same as yours. Desire says, "I am not content as I am. More money is needed; then I will be contented. More liberation is needed; then I will be contented." The quality of desire is the same, the problem of desire is the same. The problem is that the future is needed: "As I am, it is not enough; something more is needed. Whatsoever has happened to me is not enough. Something still has to happen to me; only then can I be happy." This is the nature of desire: you need more money, somebody needs a bigger house, somebody thinks of more power, politics, somebody thinks of a better wife or a better husband, somebody thinks of more education, more knowledge, somebody thinks of more miraculous powers, but it makes no difference. Desire is desire, and desirelessness is needed.

Now the paradox: if you are absolutely desireless—and in absolute desirelessness, the desire of moksha is included—a moment comes when you don't desire even moksha, you don't desire even God. You simply don't desire; you are, and there is no desire. This is the state of desirelessness. Moksha happens in this state. Moksha cannot be desired, by its very nature, because it comes only in desirelessness. Liberation cannot be desired. It cannot become a motive because it happens only when all motives have disappeared. You cannot make God an object of your desire because the desiring mind remains ungodly. The desiring mind remains unholy; the desiring mind remains worldly. When there is no desire, not even the desire for God, suddenly He has always been there. Your eyes open and you recognize Him.

Desires function as barriers. And the last desire, the most subtle desire, is the desire to be liberated. The last, subtle desire is the desire to be desireless.

> *One who is able to maintain a constant state of*
> *desirelessness, even towards the most exalted states*
> *of enlightenment, and is able to exercise the highest*
> *kind of discrimination . . .*

Of course, the ultimate in discrimination will be needed. You will have to be aware—so much so that this very, very deep desire of becoming free of all misery, of becoming free of all bondage, even

this desire does not arise. Your awareness is so perfect that not
even a small corner is left dark inside your being. You are full of
light, illuminated with awareness. That's why when Buddha is
asked again and again, "What happens to a man who becomes
enlightened?" he remains silent. He never answers. Again and
again he is asked, "Why don't you answer?" He says, "If I answer,
you will create a desire for it, and that will become a barrier. Let
me keep quiet. Let me remain silent so I don't give you a new
object for desire. If I say, 'It is *satchitananda:* it is truth, it is
consciousness, it is bliss,' immediately a desire will arise in you. If I
talk about that ecstatic state of being in God, immediately your
greed takes it. Suddenly, a desire starts arising in you. Your mind
starts saying, 'Yes, you have to seek it, you have to find it. This has
to be searched. Whatsoever the cost, but you have to become
blissful.' " Buddha says, "I don't say anything about it, because
whatsoever I say, your mind will jump on it and make a desire out
of it, and that will become the cause, and you will never be able to
attain it."

Buddha insisted that there is no moksha. He insisted that when a
man becomes aware, he simply disappears. He disappears as when
you blow out a lamp and the light disappears. The word 'nirvana'
simply means blowing a lamp out. Then you don't ask where the
flame has gone, what has happened to the flame; it simply
disappears—annihilated. Buddha insisted that there is nothing left;
when you have become enlightened everything disappears, like the
flame of a lamp put out. Why?—looks very negative—but he does
not want to give you an object of desire. Then people started
asking, "Then why should we try for such a state? It is better then
to be in the world. At least we are; miserable—but at least we are;
in anguish—but we are. And your state of nothingness has no
appeal for us."

In India, Buddhism disappeared; in China, in Burma, in Ceylon,
in Japan, it reappeared, but it never appeared in its purity again
because Buddhists learned a lesson: that man lives through desire.
If they insist that there is nothing beyond enlightenment and
everything disappears, then people are not going to follow them.
Then everything will remain as it is; only their religion will disap-
pear. So they learned a trick, and in Japan, in China, in Ceylon, in
Burma, they started talking of beautiful states after enlightenment.
They betrayed Buddha. The purity was lost; then religion spread.
Buddhism became one of the great religions of the world. They
learned the politics of the human mind. They fulfilled your desire.
They said, "Yes ... lands of tremendous beauty, Buddha-lands,

heavenly lands where eternal bliss reigns." They started talking in
positive terms. Again people's greeds were inflamed, desire arose.
People started following Buddhism, but Buddhism lost its beauty.
Its beauty was in its insistence that it would not give you any
object for desire.

Patanjali has written the best that it is possible to write about
the ultimate truth, but no religion has arisen around him, no
established church exists around him. Such a great teacher, such a
great Master has remained really without a following. Not a single
temple is devoted to him. What happened? His *Yoga Sutras* are
read, commented upon, but nothing like Christianity, Buddhism,
Jainism, Hinduism, Mohammedanism, exists with Patanjali.
Why?—because he will not give any hope to you. He will not give
any help to your desire.

*One who is able to maintain a constant state of
desirelessness, even towards the most exalted states
of enlightenment, and is able to exercise the highest
kind of discrimination, enters the state known as 'the
cloud which showers virtue'.*

Dharma megha samadhi: this word has to be understood. It is
very complex. And so many commentaries have been written on
Patanjali, but it seems they go on missing the point. *Dharma megha
samadhi* means: a moment comes when every desire has disappeared. When even the self is no more desired, when death is not
feared, virtue showers on you—as if a cloud gathers around your
head, and a beautiful shower of virtue, a benediction, a great
blessing. . . . But why does Patanjali call it 'cloud'?—one has to go
even beyond that; it is still a cloud. Before, your eyes were full of
vice, now your eyes are full of virtue, but you are still blind. Before,
nothing but misery was showering on you, just a hell was showering on you; now, you have entered heaven and everything is
perfectly beautiful, there is nothing to complain about, but still it is
a cloud. Maybe it is a white cloud, not a black cloud, but still it is a
cloud—and one has to go beyond it also. That's why he calls it
'cloud'.

That is the last barrier, and of course it is very beautiful because
it is of virtue. It is like golden chains studded with diamonds. They
are not like ordinary chains; they look very ornamental. They are
more like ornaments than chains. One would like to cling to them.
Who would not like to have a tremendous happiness showering on

oneself, a non-ending happiness? Who would not like to be in this ecstasy forever and ever? But this too is a cloud—white, beautiful, but still the real sky is hidden behind it.

There is a possibility from this exalted point to still fall back. If you become too attached to *dharma megha samadhi*, if you become too much attached, you start enjoying it too much and you don't discriminate that "I am also not this," there is a possibility that you will come back.

In Christianity, Judaism, Mohammedanism, only two states exist: hell and heaven. This is what Christians call heaven, what Patanjali calls *dharma megha samadhi*. In the West, no religion has risen beyond that. In India we have three terms: hell, heaven and moksha. Hell is absolute misery; heaven is absolute happiness; moksha is beyond both: neither hell nor heaven. In Western language, there exists not a single term equivalent to moksha. Christianity stops at heaven—*dharma megha samadhi*. Who bothers anymore to go beyond it? It is so beautiful. And you have lived in so much misery for so long; you would like to remain there forever and ever. But Patanjali says, "If you cling to it, you slip from the last rung of the ladder. You were just close to home. One step more, and then you would have achieved the point of no return—but you slipped. You were just reaching home and you missed the path. You were just at the door—a knock and the doors would have opened—but you thought that the porch was the palace and you started living there." Sooner or later you will even lose the porch, because the porch exists for those who are going into the palace. It cannot be made an abode. If you make an abode of it, sooner or later you will be thrown out: you are not worthy. You are like a beggar who has started to live on somebody's porch.

You have to enter the palace; then the porch will remain available. But if you stop at the porch even the porch will be taken away. And the porch is very beautiful, and we have never known anything like that, so certainly we misunderstand—we think the palace has come. We have lived always in anxiety, misery, tension, and even the porch, even to be close to the ultimate palace, to be so close to the ultimate truth, is so silent, so peaceful, so blissful, such a great benediction, that you cannot imagine that better than that is possible. You would like to settle here.

Patanjali says, "Remain aware." That's why he calls it a cloud. It can blind you; you can be lost in it. If you can transcend this cloud—*tatah klesa-karma-nivrttih*—*then follows freedom from afflictions and karmas.*

If you can transcend *dharma megha samadhi*, if you can transcend this heavenly state, this paradise, then only . . . then follows
freedom from afflictions and karmas. Otherwise, you will fall back
into the world. Have you seen small children play a game called
ludo, ladders and snakes? From the ladders they go on rising, and
from the snakes they go on coming back. From point ninety-nine, if
they reach a hundred they have won the game, they are victorious.
But from point ninety-nine there is a snake. If you reach ninety-
nine, you are suddenly back, back into the world.

Dharma megha samadhi is the ninety-ninth point, but the snake
is there. Before the snake takes hold of you, you have to jump to the
hundredth point. Only then, there is abode. You have come back
home; a full circle.

Then follows freedom from afflictions and karmas.

*That which can be known through the mind is very
little compared with the infinite knowledge obtained
in enlightenment, when the veils, distortions, and
impurities are removed.*

Just a few sutras back, Patanjali said that the mind is infinitely
knowledgeable, the mind can know infinitely. Now he says that
that which can be known through the mind is very little compared
with the infinite knowledge obtained in enlightenment.

As you progress higher, each state is bigger than the first state
that you have transcended. When one is lost in his senses, the mind
functions in a crippled way. When one is no more lost in the senses
and no more attached to the body, the mind starts functioning in a
perfectly healthy way. An infinite apprehension happens to mind; it
becomes capable of knowing infinities. But that too is nothing
compared to when mind is completely dropped and you start
functioning without mind. No medium is now needed. All wheels
disappear and you are immediate to reality. Not even mind is there
as an agent, as a go-between. Nothing is in between. You and the
reality are one. The knowledge that comes through mind is nothing
compared to the knowledge that happens through enlightenment.

*Having fulfilled their object, the process of change in
the three gunas comes to an end.*

For the enlightened person the whole world stops, because now there is no need for the world to go on. The ultimate has been achieved. The world exists as a situation. The world exists for your growth. The school exists for learning. When you have learned the lesson, the school is no more for you; you have graduated. When somebody attains enlightenment, he has graduated from the world. Now the school no longer has any function for him. Now he can forget about the school, and the school can forget about him. He has gone beyond, he has grown. The situation is no longer needed.

The world is a situation: it is a situation for you to go astray and come back home. It is a situation to be lost in and then come back. It is a situation to forget God and then remember Him again.

But why this situation?—because there is a subtle law: if you cannot forget God, you cannot remember Him. If there is no possibility to forget Him, how will you remember, why will you remember? That which is always available is easily forgotten. The fish in the ocean never knows the ocean, never comes across it. He lives in it, is born in it, dies in it, but never comes to know the ocean. There is only one situation when the fish comes to know the ocean: when it is taken out of the ocean. Then suddenly it becomes aware that this was the ocean, his life. When the fish is thrown on the bank, on the sand, then she knows what ocean is.

We needed to be thrown out of the ocean of God; there was no other way to know Him. The world is a great situation to become aware. Anguish is there, pain is there, but it is all meaningful. Nothing is meaningless in the world. Suffering is meaningful. The suffering is just like the fish suffering on the bank, in the sand, and making all efforts to go back to the ocean. Now, if the fish goes back to the ocean she will know. Nothing has changed—the ocean is the same, the fish is the same—but their relationship has tremendously changed. Now she will know, "This is the ocean." Now she will know how grateful she is to the ocean. The suffering has created a new understanding. Before also she was in the same ocean, but now the same ocean is no more the same because a new understanding exists, a new awareness, a new recognition.

Man needs to be thrown out of God. To be thrown into the world is nothing but to be thrown out of God. And it is out of compassion, out of the compassion of the whole that you are thrown out, so that you try to find the way back. By effort, by arduous effort you will be able to reach, and then you will understand. You have to pay for it by your efforts, otherwise God would be too cheap. And when a thing is too cheap, you cannot enjoy it. Otherwise, God would be too obvious. When a thing is too obvious you tend to forget. Otherwise, God would be too close to you and there would be no space to know Him. That will be the real misery, not to know Him. The misery of the world is not a misery; it is a blessing in disguise because only through this misery will you come to know the tremendous blissfulness of recognizing, of seeing face to face . . . the divine truth.

*Having fulfilled their object, the process of change in
the three gunas comes to an end.*

The whole world of the three gunas: *sattva, rajas, tamas,* comes to an end. Whenever somebody becomes enlightened, for him the world comes to an end. Of course, others go on dreaming. If there are too many fish suffering on the bank, in the hot sand, in the burning sun, and one fish tries and tries and jumps into the ocean, again back home, for her, or for him, the hot sun and the burning sand and all the misery has disappeared. It is already a nightmare of the past; but for others, it exists.

When a fish like Buddha, Patanjali, jumps into the ocean, for them the world has disappeared. They are again back in the cool womb of the ocean. They are back again, joined, connected to the infinite life. They are no longer disconnected; they are no longer alienated. They have become aware. They have come back with a new understanding: alert, enlightened—but for others the world continues.

These sutras of Patanjali are nothing but messages of a fish who has reached home, trying to jump and say something to the people who are still on the bank and suffering. Maybe they are very close to the ocean, just on the border, but they don't know how to enter into it. They are not making enough effort, or, are making them in the wrong directions, or, are simply lost in misery and have accepted that this is what life is, or, are so frustrated, discouraged, that they are not making any effort. Yoga is the effort to reach to that reality with which we have become disconnected. To be re-connected is to be a yogi. Yoga means: re-connection, re-union, re-merging.

*Kramaha, the process, is the succession of changes
that occur from moment to moment, which become
apprehensible at the final end of the transformations
of the three gunas.*

In this small sutra Patanjali has said everything that modern physics has come to discover. Just thirty or forty years ago, it would have been impossible to understand this sutra because the whole quantum physics is present, in seed form, in this small sutra. And this is good, because this is just the last-but-one. So Patanjali summarizes the whole world of physics in this last-but-one sutra: then, the *meta*physics. This is the essential physics. The greatest insight that has come to physics in this century is the theory of quantum.

Max Planck discovered a very unbelievable thing. He discovered that life is not a continuity; everything is discontinuous. One moment of time is separate from another moment of time, and between the two moments of time there is a space. They are not connected; they are disconnected. One atom is separate from another atom, and between the two atoms there is great space. They are not connected. This is what he calls 'quanta': distinct, separate atoms not bridged with each other, floating in infinite space, but separate—just as you pour peas from one carton into another and the peas all fall, separate, distinct, or, if you pour oil from one container into another, the oil falls in a continuity.

The existence is like peas, separate. Why does Patanjali mention this?—because he says, "One atom, another atom: these are two things the world consists of. Just between the two is the space. That is what the whole consists of, the God. Call it space, call it *Brahma*, call it *Purusa* or whatsoever you like; the world consists of distinct atoms, and the whole consists of the infinite space between the two."

Now physicists say that if we press the whole world and press the space out of it, all the stars and all the suns can be pressed into just a small ball. Only that much matter exists. It is really space. Matter is very rare, here and there. If we press the earth very much, we can put it into a matchbox. If all the space is thrown out, unbelievable! "And that too, if we go on pressing it still more," Patanjali says, "then even that small quantity will disappear." Now physicists say that when matter disappears it leaves black holes.

Everything comes out of nothingness, plays around, disappears again into nothingness. As there are material bodies: earth, sun, stars, there are, just similar to them, empty holes, black holes. Those black holes are nothingness condensed. It is not simply nothingness; it is very dynamic—whirlpools of nothingness. If a star comes by a black hole, the black hole will suck it in. So it is very dynamic, but it is nothing—no matter in it, simply absence of matter; just pure space, but tremendously powerful. It can suck any star in, and the star will disappear into nothingness; it will be reduced to nothingness. So ultimately, if we try, then all matter will disappear. It comes out of a tremendous nothingness, and it drops again into a tremendous nothingness: out of nothingness, and back into nothingness.

Kramaha, the process—the process of quantum—*is the succession of changes that occur from moment to moment which becomes apprehensible at the final end of the transformations of the three gunas.*

This the yogi comes to see at the final stage, when all the three gunas are disappearing into black holes, disappearing into nothingness. That's why yogis have called the world *maya*, a magic show.

Have you seen a magician producing a mango tree within seconds, and then it goes on growing; and not only that—within seconds mangoes have appeared ... out of nothing? It is just illusory; he creates illusion. Maybe he sends deep messages to your unconscious. It is just like deep hypnosis. He creates the idea, but he visualizes his idea so deeply and he impresses it on your unconscious so deeply that you also start seeing it as he wants you to see it. Nothing is happening. The tree is not there, the mango is not there. And it is possible, just out of great imagination, to create a mango tree, and mangoes come. Not only that, but he can pluck one mango and give it to you and you will say, "Very sweet."

Hindus call the world *maya*, a magic show. It is God's imagination. The whole is dreaming, the whole is projecting.

You go to a movie: on a wide screen you see a great story being enacted, and you see that everything seems to be continuous, but it is not. If the film is moved a little slower, you will see that everything is discontinuous—quanta. One picture goes, another comes, another goes, another comes, but between two pictures there is a gap. In that gap you can see the real screen. When the pictures are moving very fast, they create an illusion of movement. Of course, a movie film is not a moving film. It is as static a photograph as any other. The movement is illusory because those static photographs are running after each other so fast, the gap between them is so small, that you cannot see the gap. So everything looks as if it is continuous.

I move my hand: to show this hand moving in a film, thousands of pictures will be needed of each state of stasis—from this point to this, from this point to this, from this point to this. The one simple movement of the hand will be divided into thousands of small static movements. Then all those pictures move fast: the hand seems to be moving. It is an illusion. Deep down, between two pictures, it is a white screen, empty.

Patanjali says, "The world is nothing but a cinematograph, a projection." But this understanding arises only when one achieves to the last point of understanding. When he sees all gunas stopped, nothing is moving, suddenly he becomes aware that the whole story was created by illusory movement, by fast movement. This is what is happening to modern physics.

First they said when they had come to the atom, "Now this is the ultimate; it cannot be divided any more." Then they also divided the atom. Then they came to electrons: "Now it cannot be divided any more." Now they have divided that too. Now they have come to nothingness; now they don't know what has come. Division, division, division, and a point has come in modern physics where matter has completely disappeared. Modern physics has reached via matter, and Patanjali and the yogis have reached to the same point via consciousness. Up to this last-but-one sutra, physics has reached. Up to this last-but-one sutra, scientists can have an approach, an understanding, a penetration. The last sutra is not possible for scientists, because that last sutra can be achieved only if you move through consciousness, not through matter; not through objects, but directly through subjectivity.

Purusartha-sunyanam gunanam pratiprasavah
kaivalyam svarupa-pratistha va citi-sakter iti.

Kaivalya is the state of enlightenment that follows
the remergence of the gunas, due to their becoming
devoid of the object of the Purusa.

In this state, the Purusa is established in his real
nature, which is pure consciousness. Finish.

Kaivalya is the state of enlightenment that follows the remergence of the three gunas ... when the world stops, when the process, the *kramaha* of the world stops, when you become able to see between two moments of time and two atoms of matter, and you can move into space, and you can see that everything has arisen out of space and is moving back into space; when you have become so aware that suddenly the illusory world disappears like a dream, then *kaivalya*. Then you are left as pure consciousness—with no identity, with no name, no form. Then you are the purest of the pure. Then you are the most fundamental, the most essential, the most existential, and you are established in this purity, aloneness.

Patanjali says, *"Kaivalya* is the state of enlightenment that follows the remergence of the gunas, due to their becoming devoid of the object of the Purusa. In this state the Purusa is established in his real nature." You have come back home. The journey has been long, torturous, arduous, but you have come back home. The fish has jumped into the ocean which is pure consciousness. Patanjali does not say anything more about it, because more cannot be said. And when Patanjali says, "Finish; the end," he does not only mean that the *Yoga Sutras* finish here. He says, "All possibility to express ends here. All possibility to say anything about the ultimate reality ends here. Beyond this is only experience. Expression ends here." And nobody has been able to go beyond it—nobody. Not a single exception exists in the whole history of human consciousness. People have tried. Very few have even reached to where Patanjali had reached, but nobody has been able to go beyond Patanjali.

That's why I say he's the alpha and the omega. He starts from the very beginning; nobody has been able to find a better beginning than him. He begins from the very beginning and he comes to the very end. When he says, "Finish," he's simply saying expression is finished, definition is finished, description is finished. If you have really come with him up to now, there is only experience beyond. Now starts the existential. One can be it, but one cannot say it. One can live in it, but one cannot define it. Words won't help. All language is impotent beyond this point. Simply saying this much: that one achieves to one's own true nature—Patanjali stops. That's the goal: to know one's nature and to live in it—because unless we reach to our own natures we will be in misery. All misery is indicative that we are living somehow unnaturally. All misery is simply symptomatic that somehow our nature is not being fulfilled, that somehow we are not in tune with our reality. The misery is not your enemy; it is just a symptom. It indicates. It is like a thermometer; it simply shows that you are going wrong somewhere. Put it all right, put yourself right; bring yourself in harmony, come back, tune yourself. When every misery disappears one is in tune with one's nature. That nature Lao Tzu calls *tao*, Patanjali calls *kaivalya*, Mahavir calls *moksha*, Buddha calls *nirvana*. But whatsoever you want to call it—it has no name and it has no form—it is in you, present, right this moment. You have lost the ocean because

you have come out of your self. You have moved too much in the
outer world. Move inwards. Now, let this be your pilgrimage: move
inwards.

It happened: A Sufi mystic, Bayazid, was going on a pilgrimage
to Mecca. It was difficult. He was poor and somehow he had
managed the travelling expenses by begging for years. Now he was
very happy. He had almost the necessary money to go to Mecca,
and then he travelled. By the time he reached near Mecca, just
outside the town he met a fakir, his Master. He was sitting there
just under a tree, and he said, "Oh fool, where are you going?"
Bayazid looked at him; he had never seen such a luminous being.
He came near him and the man said, "Give me whatsoever you
have! Where are you going?" He said, "I am going to Mecca for a
pilgrimage." He said, "Finish. There is now no need; you just
worship me. You can move around me as many times as you like.
You can do your *parikrama*, your circumlocution, around me. I am
Mecca." And Bayazid was so filled with this person's magnetism
that he gave all his money, he worshipped. Then the old man said,
"Now go back home"; and he went back home.

When he went into his town people gathered and said, "Something seems to have happened to you. So really it works, going to
Mecca works? You are looking luminous, so full of light." He said,
"Stop this nonsense! One old man met me—he changed my whole
pilgrimage. He says, 'Go home,' and since then I have been going
home, inwards. I have arrived. I have arrived, I have reached to my
Mecca."

The outer Mecca is not the real Mecca. The real Mecca is inside
you. You are the temple of God. You are the abode of the ultimate.
So the question is not where to find truth, the question is: how have
you lost it? The question is not where to go; you are already
there—stop going.

Drop from all the paths. All paths are of desire, extensions of
desire, projections of desire: going somewhere, going somewhere,
always somewhere else, never here.

Seeker, leave all paths, because all paths lead there, and He is
here.

Purusartha-sunyanam gunanam pratiprasavah
kaivalyam svarupa-pratistha va citi-sakter iti.

CHAPTER TEN
May 10, 1976

I AM IN FAVOR
OF LOVE

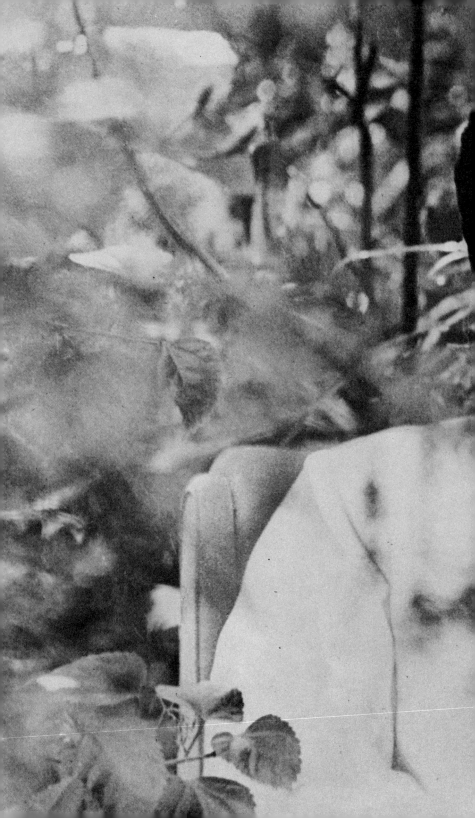

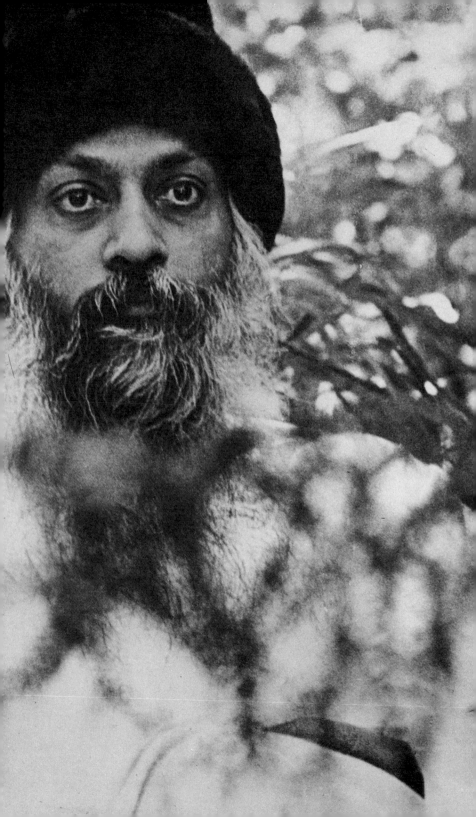

The first question:

Why is every human being full of problems and unhappy?

THE FIRST THING: BECAUSE MAN CAN BE TREMEN-
DOUSLY HAPPY, the possibility exists, hence, his unhappiness. Nobody else—no animal, no bird, no tree, no
rock—can be so happy as man. The possibility, the tremendous possibility that you can be happy, eternally happy, that
you can be at the top of a bliss mountain, creates unhappiness. And
when you see around you, you are just in the valley, a dark valley,
and you could have been at the top of the peak: the comparison, the
possibility, and the actuality.

If you were not born to be Buddhas, then there would be no
unhappiness. So, the more perceptive a person is, the more unhappy. The more sensitive a person is, the more unhappy. The more
alert a person is, the more he feels the sadness, the more he feels
the potentiality and the contradiction, that nothing is happening
and he's stuck.

Man is unhappy because man can be tremendously happy. And
unhappiness is not bad. It is the very drive that will take you to the
peak. If you are not unhappy, then you will not move. If you are not
unhappy in your dark valley, why should you make any effort to
climb uphill? It is going to be arduous—unless the sun shining at
the top becomes a challenge, unless the very existence of the top
creates a mad urge to reach, unless the very possibility provokes
you to seek and search. People who are not very alert, sensitive, are
not very unhappy. Have you seen any idiot unhappy?—impossible.
An idiot cannot be unhappy because he cannot be aware of the
possibility that he is carrying within himself.

You are conscious that you are a seed, and the tree can happen.
It is just by the corner. The goal is not very far away; that makes
you unhappy. It is a good indication. To feel unhappiness deeply is
the first step. Certainly, Buddha feels it more than you. That's why
he renounced the valley and he started climbing uphill. Small
things that you come across every day became great provocations
for him. Seeing a man ill, seeing an old man leaning on his staff,
seeing a dead body, was enough; that very night he left his palace.

He became aware of where he was: "The same is going to happen to me. Sooner or later, I will become ill and old and dead, so what is the point of being here? Before the opportunity is taken away from me, I should attain to something which is eternal." A great desire arose in him to reach to the peak. That peak we call God; that peak we call *kaivalya*, that peak we call *moksha, nirvana;* but that peak exists within you like a seed. It has to unfold. So great sensitive souls suffer more. Idiots don't suffer, dullards don't suffer. They are already happy in their ordinary life: earning a little money, making a small house—finished. Their whole possibility is only that.

If you are aware that this can't be the goal, this can't be the destiny, then a great suffering will enter into your being like a sharp sword. It will penetrate to the very core of your being. A great scream will arise in your heart and that will be the beginning of a new life, of a new style of life, of a new foundation of life.

So, the first thing I would like to say is: to feel unhappy is blissful; to feel unhappy is a blessing. Not to feel so is to be dull.

The second thing: human beings remain in misery because they go on creating misery for themselves.

So first, understand it. To be unhappy is good, but I am not saying that you should go on creating your unhappiness more and more. I am saying: it is good because it provokes you to go beyond it. But go beyond it, otherwise it is no good.

People go on creating their pattern of misery. There is a reason: the mind resists change. The mind is very orthodox. It wants to continue on the old path, because the old is known. If you are born a Hindu, you will die a Hindu. If you are born a Christian, you will die a Christian. People don't change. A particular ideology becomes so ingrained in you that you become afraid to change it. You feel apprehensive because with this you are familiar. The new—who knows?—may not even be so good as the old. And the old is known; you are well acquainted with it. Maybe it is miserable, but at least it is familiar. On each step, every moment of life you are deciding something, whether you know it or not. The decision encounters you every moment—whether to follow the old path that you have been following up to now, or to choose the new. At every step the road bifurcates. And there are two types of people. Those who choose the well-trodden path; of course, they move in a circle. They choose the known, and the known is a circle. They have known it already. They choose their future just as it has been in their past. They move in a circle. They go on making their past their future. No growth happens. They are simply repeating; they are automata, robot-like.

Then there is another type of person, type of awareness, who is always alert to choose the new. Maybe the new creates more suffering, maybe the new leads astray, but at least it is new. It will not be just a repetition of the past. The new has the possibility of learning, growth, of the potential becoming actual.

So remember, whenever there is to be a choice, choose the untrodden path. But you have been taught just the contrary. You have been taught always to choose the known. You have been taught to be very clever and cunning. Of course, there are comforts with the known. One comfort is that you can remain unconscious with the known. There is no need to be conscious. If you are following the same path you can move almost asleep, like a somnambulist. If you are coming back to your own home, and every day you have been coming, you need not be aware; you can just come unconsciously. When it is time to turn to the right, you turn; there is no need to keep any alertness. That's why people like to follow the old path: no need to be aware. And awareness is one of the most difficult things to achieve. Whenever you are moving in a new direction, you have to be aware at each step.

Choose the new. It will give you awareness. It is not going to be comfortable. Growth is never comfortable; growth is painful. Growth goes through suffering. You pass through fire, but only then you become pure gold. Then all that is not gold is burnt, reduced to ashes. Only the purest remains in you. You have been taught to follow the old because on the old you will be committing less mistakes. But you will commit the basic mistake, and the basic mistake will be this: that growth happens only when you remain available to the new, with the possibility of committing new mistakes. Of course, there is no need to repeat an old mistake again and again, but be capable and courageous for committing new mistakes—because each new mistake makes a learning, becomes a learning situation. Each time you go astray, you have to find the path back home. And this going and coming, this constant forgetting and remembering, creates an integration within your being.

Always choose the new; even if it looks worse than the old I say, always choose the new. It looks inconvenient—choose the new. It is uncomfortable, insecure—choose the new. It is not a question of 'new'; it is to give you an opportunity to be more aware. Efficiency has been taught to you as the goal. It is not. Alertness is the goal. Efficiency makes you follow the old path again and again, because you will be more efficient on the old path. You will know all the nooks and corners. You have travelled on it for so many years, or maybe so many lives; you will be more and more efficient. But efficiency is not the goal. Efficiency is the goal for a mechanism. A machine has to be efficient, but a man?—man is not a machine. A man has to be more aware, and if efficiency comes out of awareness, good, beautiful. If it comes at the cost of awareness you are committing a great sin against life, and then you will remain unhappy. And this unhappiness will become a pattern. You will simply move in a vicious circle. One unhappiness will lead you to another, and so on and so forth.

Unhappiness as an awareness is a blessing, but unhappiness as a style of life is a curse. Don't make it your style of life. I see many people have made it their style of life. They don't know any other style of life. Even if you say to them, they won't listen. They will go on asking why they are unhappy, and they won't listen that they are creating their unhappiness every moment. That's the meaning of the theory of karma.

The theory of karma simply says that whatsoever is happening to you is your doing. Somewhere, on an unconscious level, you must be creating it—because nothing happens to you from the outside. Everything bubbles from the inside. If you are sad, you must be creating your sadness somewhere in your innermost being. From there it comes. You must be manufacturing it somewhere within your soul. Watch: if you are miserable, meditate on your misery, on how you create it. You always ask, "Who is responsible for misery?" Nobody is responsible except you. The mind goes on saying to you that if you are a husband, your wife is creating your misery. If you are a wife, your husband is creating your misery. If you are poor, the rich are creating your misery. It always goes on throwing responsibility on somebody else.

This has to be a very fundamental understanding: that except you, nobody is responsible. Once you understand it things start changing. If you are creating your misery and you love it, then go on creating. Then don't create a problem out of it. It is nobody's business to interfere with you. If you want to be sad, you love to be sad, be perfectly sad. But if you don't want to be sad, then there is no need—don't create. Watch how you create your misery: what is the pattern?—how have you managed it inside? People are continuously creating their moods. You go on throwing the responsibility on others; then you will never change. Then you will remain miserable, because what can you do? If others are creating, what can you do? Unless others change, nothing is in your hands. By throwing responsibility on others, you become a slave. Take the responsibility into your own hands.

A few days ago a sannyasin told me that her husband has always been creating problems for her. And when she tells her story it will look, apparently, that of course the husband is responsible. She has eight children from the husband, and then the husband has three more children from another woman, and one child from his secretary. He has been continuously fooling around with any woman that comes along. Of course, anybody will sympathize with this poor woman. She has suffered a lot, and the game continues. The husband is not earning much. The woman, the wife, earns, and she has to pay for these children which he has brought into the world from other women also. Of course, she is in a great misery, but who is responsible? I told her, "If you are really in misery, why should you continue to be with this man? Drop out. You should have dropped out long before. There is no need to continue." And she understood, which is a rare thing—very late, very delayed, but still not too late. Still, her life is there. Now if she insists that she would like to remain with this man, then she is insisting for her own misery. Then she is enjoying the misery trip. Then she is enjoying condemning the husband; then she is enjoying attracting sympathy from everybody else. And of course, with whomsoever she will come in contact, they will sympathize with the poor woman.

Never ask for sympathy. Ask for understanding, but never ask for sympathy. Otherwise, sympathy can be such a good pay-off that you would like to remain miserable. Then you have some investment in your misery. If you are no more miserable, people won't sympathize with you. Have you watched?—nobody sympathizes with a happy man. It is something absolutely absurd. People should sympathize with the happy man, but nobody sympathizes. In fact, people feel antagonistic to a happy man. In fact, to be happy is very dangerous. To be happy, and express your happiness, you are putting yourself in very great danger—everybody will be your enemy, because everybody will feel, "How come I am unhappy and you have become happy? Impossible! This cannot be allowed. This is too much."

In a society which is unhappy and consists of miserable people, a happy person is a stranger. That's why we poisoned Socrates, we killed Jesus, we crucified Mansur. We have never been at ease with happy people. Somehow, they hurt our egos very much. People crucified Jesus; when he was alive they killed him. He was very young, only thirty-three. He had not yet seen the whole life. He was just beginning his life, just a bud was opening, and people killed him because he was too much to tolerate. So happy?—everybody

was hurt. They killed this man. And then they started worshipping
him. Just see ... now they have been worshipping him for two
thousand years, crucified. But with a crucified Jesus you can sympathize; with a happy Jesus you feel antagonistic.

The same is happening here. I am a happy man. If you want me
to be worshipped, you will have to manage for a crucifixion. There
is no other way. Then people who are against me will become my
followers. But first they will have to see me on the cross, not before
it. Nobody has ever worshipped a happy man. First, the happy man
has to be destroyed. Then, of course, he is manageable. Now you
can sympathize with Jesus. Whenever you see, tears start flowing
into your eyes: "Poor man; how much he suffered." A dancing
Christ creates trouble.

In Sweden, a man is trying to make a film on Jesus: *Jesus the
Man*. For ten years he has been trying, but a thousand and one
barriers: the government won't allow—"Jesus the man?—no!" Because 'Jesus the man' means that this man may have been in love
with Mary Magdalene, and the man will bring it out. Jesus loved
women. It is natural; nothing is wrong in it. He was a happy man.
He sometimes loved wine also. He was a man who could celebrate.
Now, Jesus the man is dangerous. And this man wants to make a
film on Jesus the man; not the son of God, but the son of man. This
will be troublesome. And if he starts working out a story, he will
have to bring in some illegal love affair with Mary, because a virgin
woman cannot give birth. Jesus was not the son of Joseph; that
much is certain. But he must have been the son of somebody. The
government is against, the church is against: "You are trying to
prove Jesus a bastard! Impossible! The film cannot be allowed."
And Jesus loving the prostitute Mary Magdalene?—and certainly,
he loved. He was a happy man. Love simply happens around a
happy man. He enjoyed life. It is a God-given blessing; one has to
enjoy it. Every religious man is a celebrating soul.

Then they killed this man, crucified him, and since then they
have been worshipping him. Now he is manageable; he creates
much sympathy in you. Jesus on the cross is more attractive than
Buddha sitting under the Bodhi tree. Jesus on the cross is more
attractive than Krishna playing his flute. Jesus became the world
religion. Krishna?—who bothers about him? Even Hindus feel a
little guilty about sixteen thousand women dancing around him—
"Impossible, it is just a myth." Hindus say it is beautiful poetry,
and they go on interpreting. They say, "These sixteen thousand
women were not really women; these are sixteen thousand *nadis*,

the nervous system, the sixteen thousand nerves in the human body. It is a symbolic expression about the human body. Krishna is the soul, and sixteen thousand nerves are the Gopis dancing around the soul." Then everything is okay. But if they are real women, then it is difficult, very difficult to accept.

Jainas, another religion of India, have thrown Krishna into hell because of these sixteen thousand women. In the Jain *Puranas*, they say, "Krishna is in the seventh hell, the last ... and he will not be coming up soon. He will be there up to the moment this whole creation is destroyed. He will come up only when the next creation starts; millions and millions of years still to wait. He has committed a great sin"; and the great sin is because he was celebrating. The great sin is because he was dancing.

Mahavir is more acceptable, Buddha still more acceptable. Krishna seems to be a renegade who betrayed the serious people. He was non-serious, happy; not sombre, not a long-face—laughing, dancing. And that is the true way. I would like to say to you, dance your way to God, laugh your way to God. Don't go with serious faces. God is already much too bored with that type.

Sympathy is a great investment, and that can be continued only if you can go on getting sympathy, only if you remain miserable. So if one misery stops, you create another; if one illness leaves you, you create another. Watch it—you are playing a very dangerous game with yourself. That's why people are miserable and unhappy. Otherwise, there is no need.

Put all your energy into being happy, and don't bother about others. Your happiness is your destiny; nobody is entitled to interfere with it. But the society goes on interfering; it is a vicious circle. You were born, and of course you were born into a society already there, a given society of neurotic people, of people who are all miserable and unhappy. Your parents, your family, your society, your country, are already there waiting for you. And a small child is born; the whole society jumps on the child, starts culturing him, cultivating him. It is as if a child is born in a madhouse, and all the mad people start cultivating. Of course, they have to help—the child is so small and does not know anything about the world. They will teach whatsoever they know. They will enforce whatsoever has been enforced on them by their parents, by other mad people. Have you seen that whenever a child starts giggling and laughing, something in you becomes uneasy? You immediately want to tell him, "Shut up and suck your lollipop!" Immediately, something in you says, "Shut up!" When a child starts giggling, do you feel jealous, or what? You cannot allow a child running hither and thither, jumping, just sheer joy.

I have heard about two American women, two spinsters. They visited Italy to see an old church. American visitors! In the church they saw an Italian woman praying, and her four or five children running inside the church and making much noise, and simply happy, completely oblivious that it was a church. Those two American women could not tolerate it: "This is too much. This is sacrilege." They went up to the woman who was praying, the mother, and told her, "These children are yours? This is a church and some discipline should be maintained! They should be controlled." The woman, with prayerful eyes, tears flowing and tremendously happy, looked at them and said, "This is their Father's house, can't they play here?" But this attitude is rare, very rare.

Humanity is dominated by mad people: politicians, priests, they are mad because ambition is madness—and they go on enforcing their pattern. When a child is born he is a bubbling energy, an infinite source of bliss, happiness, joy, delight; sheer delight, nothing else—overflowing. You start controlling him: you start cutting his limbs, you start butchering him. You say, "There are proper times to laugh." Proper times to laugh?—that means proper times to be alive? You are saying the same thing: proper times to be alive—"You should not be alive twenty-four hours." There are proper times to cry. But when a child feels like laughing what is he supposed to do? He has to control, and when you control your laughter it goes bitter and sour within you. The energy that was going out has been held back. Holding back the energy, you become stuck. The child wanted to reach out, to run around, to jump and jog and dance; now he is stopped. His energy is ready to overflow, but by and by he learns only one thing: to freeze his energy. That's why so many stuck people are in the world, so uptight, continuously controlling. They cannot cry; tears are too unmanly. They cannot laugh; laughter seems to be too uncivilized. Life is denied, death is worshipped. You would like a child to behave like an old man, and old people start forcing their deaths on new generations.

I have heard about an old woman of ninety, a countess, who had a very big house with acres of greenery. She came one day to look around the property; it was very big. Just beyond the pond, behind the woods, she saw two young people making love. She asked the driver, "What are these people doing here?"—ninety years of age; she may have forgotten ... "What are these people doing here?" The driver had to say the truth. Very politely he said, "They are

making love. They are young people." The old lady was very much
annoyed and she said, "Does such a thing still go on in the world?"
When you become old, do you think the whole world has become
old? When you are dying, do you think the whole world is dying?
The world goes on renewing itself, reviving itself. That's why it
takes the old people away, and gives small babies back to the
world. It turns the old people into small babies.

Existence goes on peopling the earth with new people. Whenever
it sees that a person has gone completely stuck—now there is no
more flow, no more juice, and the person is simply shrinking and
unnecessarily becoming a burden on earth—then life removes him.
The person goes back into the existence, is destroyed. The earth
goes to the earth, the sky goes to the sky, the air to the air, the fire
to the fire, the water to the water. Then out of that earth, out of that
water and fire a new baby is born—flowing, young, fresh, ready to
live and dance again. Just as flowers come to the tree, just as the
tree flowers, the earth goes on babying, goes on creating new babies.

If you really want to be happy you have to remain young, alive,
available to crying, laughter, available to all dimensions, flowing all
over, streaming. Then you will remain happy. But remember, you
will not get any sympathy. People may throw rocks at you, but that
is worth it. People may think that you are irreligious, they may
condemn you, they may call names to you, but don't be worried
about it. It doesn't matter. The only thing that matters is your
happiness.

And you have to undo many things; only then can you become
happy. Whatsoever has been done by the society has to be undone.
Wherever you are stuck—you were going to laugh and your father
looked at you with anger and said, "Stop!"—you will have to start
again from there. Tell your father, "Please, now I am going to again
start laughing." Somewhere inside your head your father is still
holding you: "Stop!" Have you watched? If you meditate deeply
you will come to see and hear your parental voices within. You
were going to cry and the mother stopped you, and of course you
were helpless and you had to compromise to survive. There was no
other way. You had to depend on these people and they had their
conditions; otherwise, they wouldn't give you milk, they wouldn't
give you food, they wouldn't give you any support. And how can a
small child exist without the support? He has to compromise. He
says, "Okay. Just to survive, I will follow whatsoever you say." So
by and by, he becomes false. By and by, he goes against himself. He
wanted to laugh but the father was not allowing it, so he kept quiet.
By and by, he becomes a pretender, a hypocrite.

And a hypocrite can never be happy, because happiness is being true to your life-energy. Happiness is a function of being true. Happiness is not somewhere, that you go and purchase it. Happiness is not awaiting you somewhere, that you have to find the path and reach it. No, happiness is a function of being true, authentic. Whenever you are true, you are happy. Whenever you are untrue, you are unhappy.

And I will not say to you that if you are untrue you will be unhappy in your next life, no. This is all nonsense. If you are untrue, right now you are unhappy. Watch—whenever you are untrue, you feel uneasiness, unhappiness, because the energy is not flowing. The energy is not river-like; it is stuck, dead, frozen. And you would like to flow. Life is flow; death is frozenness. Unhappiness comes because many of your parts are frozen. They were never allowed to function and, by and by, you have learned the trick to control them. Now you have even forgotten that you are controlling something. You have lost your roots in the body. You have lost your roots in the truth of your body.

People are living like ghosts; that's why they are miserable. When I see inside you, rarely do I come across an alive man. People have become like ghosts, phantoms. You are not in your body; you are somewhere about your head hovering like a ghost, just like a balloon around the head. Just a small thread is joining you to the body. That thread keeps you alive, that's all, but it is not a delight. You will have to become conscious, you will have to meditate, and you will have to drop all the controls. You will have to unlearn, undo, and then for the first time you will again become flowing.

Of course, discipline is needed, not as control but as awareness. A controlled discipline is a deadening phenomenon. When you are alert, aware, a discipline comes easily out of that awareness—not that you force it, not that you plan it. No, moment to moment your awareness decides how to respond. And an alert person responds in such a way that he remains happy, and he does not create unhappiness for others.

That's all religion is all about: remain happy, and don't create any situation for anybody to be unhappy. If you can help, make others happy. If you cannot, then at least make yourself happy.

The second question:

I keep on dreaming that I am flying. What is happening?

G.K. Chesterton has said, "The angels fly because they take themselves lightly."

That must be happening to you; you must be becoming an angel. Allow it. The more light you feel, the more happy you feel, the less will be the pull of gravitation. Gravitation makes graves out of you. Heaviness is a sin. To be heavy simply means that you are loaded with unlived experiences, incomplete experiences; that you are loaded with much junk, unfinished. You wanted to love a woman but it was difficult, because Mahatma Gandhi is against it; it is difficult because Vivekanand is against it; it is difficult because all the great seers and sages go on propounding *brahmacharya*, celibacy. You wanted to love, but all the sages were against it, so you somehow controlled yourself. Now that is like a junk load on you. If you ask me, I will say you should have loved. Even now, nothing is lost; you should love. Complete it. I know the seers and sages are right, but I don't say that you are wrong.

And let me explain the paradox to you. The seers and sages are right, but they come to this understanding after they have loved much, after they have lived, after they have experienced all that love implies. Then they come to understanding, and *brahmacharya* flowers. It is not against love, it is through love that *brahmacharya* flowers. Now you are reading books, scriptures, and through the scriptures you go on getting ideas. Those ideas cripple you. Those ideas are not wrong in themselves, but you take them from the books, and the sages come to them through their own lives. Just go back into history, in the old *Puranas*, and see your sages: they loved much, they lived much; they lived tremendously human lives with power, intensity. And then, by and by, they came to understand.

It is only life that brings understanding. You wanted to be angry but all the scriptures are against it, so you never allowed anger. Now that anger goes on accumulating—piles upon piles—and you are carrying that load, almost crushed under it. That's why you feel so heavy. Throw it out, drop it! Go into an empty room and be angry, and be *really* angry; beat the pillow, and do things to the walls, and talk to the walls and say things that you always wanted to say but you have not said. Be in a rage, explode, and you will come to a beautiful experience. After the explosion, after the storm, a silence will come to you, will pervade you, a silence that has never been known by you, an unburdening. You may suddenly feel light!

Vidya has asked this question. I can see that she is feeling light. Go deeper into it so that not only in dreams, but *actually* you can fly.

If you are not carrying the past, you have such a lightness—feather-like. You live but you don't touch the earth. You live but you don't leave any footprints on the earth. You live but nothing is scratched by you, and a grace surrounds your life, your being—an aura, a glow. It is not only that you will be light, but whosoever will come in contact with you will suddenly be filled by something so graceful, so beautiful. Flowers will shower around you, and you will have a fragrance that is not of this earth. But that happens only when you are unburdened.

Mahavira has called this unburdening *nirjara*—dropping everything. But how to drop? You have been taught not to be angry. I also teach you how not to be angry, but I don't say to you not to be angry. I say: be angry. No need to be angry on someone, with someone; that complicates. Just be angry in a vacuum. Go to the river where there is nobody and simply be angry, and do whatsoever you feel like doing. After a great catharsis of anger you will fall down on the sand, and you will see that you are flying. The past has, for a moment, disappeared.

And this same has to be done to every emotion. You will feel, by and by, that if you try to be angry, you will pass through a sequence of emotions. First you will get angry, then suddenly you will start crying, out of nowhere. Anger relaxed, released—another layer of your being is touched, another load of sadness. Behind each anger there is sadness, because whenever you withhold your anger you become sad. So after each layer of anger, there is a layer of sadness. When anger is released, you will feel sad. Release that sadness—you will start crying, sobbing. Sob, cry, let tears flow. Nothing is wrong in them. Tears are one of the most beautiful things in the world: so relaxing, so relieving. And when the tears have gone, suddenly you will see another emotion: a smile is spreading somewhere deep within you, because whenever sadness is released, one starts feeling happy, a very smooth, delicate happiness, fragile. It will come up, it will bubble and it will spread all over your being. And then you will see that you are laughing for the first time—a belly laugh, like Swami Sardar Gurdayal Singh; a belly laugh. Learn from him. He is our Zorba the Greek in this ashram. Learn from him how to laugh.

Unless your belly goes into ripples you are not laughing. People laugh from the head; they should laugh from the belly. After sadness is released, you will see a laughter arising, almost maddening; a mad laughter. You are as if possessed and you laugh loudly. And after laughter has gone, you will feel light, weightless, flying. First it will appear in your dreams, and by and by, in your awakened state of being also you will feel that you are no longer walking, you are flying.

Yes, Chesterton is right: angels fly because they take themselves lightly.

Take yourself lightly.

Ego takes itself very seriously. Now, there is a problem: egoistic people become very much interested in religion. And in fact, they are almost incapable of being religious. Only people who are non-serious can become religious, but they are not too interested in religion. So a paradox, a problem exists in the world. Serious people, ill people, sad people—uptight, hung-up in their heads—they become very much interested in religion because religion gives them their greatest ego-trip. They are doing something other-worldly, and the whole world is just worldly—materialists, condemned. Everybody is going to hell; only these religious people are going to heaven. They feel very, very strengthened in their egos. But these are the people who cannot become religious. These are the people who have destroyed all the religions of the world.

Whenever a Buddha arises, these people start gathering. While he is alive he does not allow them to become powerful. But when he is gone, by and by, the serious people start manipulating the non-serious people. That's how all the religions become organized, and all religions become dead. While Buddha is there, he goes on spreading his smile, and he goes on helping people.

So many times I have told the story: that Buddha comes one day with a flower in his hand, and sits silently. Minutes pass; then the hour is passing and everybody is worried, uncomfortable, uneasy: "Why is he not speaking?" He has never done that before. And he goes on looking at the flower as if he has completely forgotten the thousands of people who have gathered to listen to him. And then one disciple, Mahakashyap, starts laughing, a belly laugh. Amidst that hushed silence his laughter spreads. Buddha looks at him. He calls him close, gives him the flower and says, "Whatsoever I could say through words I have told to you, and whatsoever I cannot say through the words, I transfer it to Mahakashyap"—to a laughing Mahakashyap. To laughter Buddha gives his heritage? But Mahakashyap disappears. Those serious people who could not understand became the manipulators. When Buddha is gone, nobody hears anything about Mahakashyap. But what happened to Mahakashyap, to whom Buddha had given the most secret message: that which cannot be delivered through words, that which can only be delivered and received in silence and laughter, that which can only be given by tremendous silence to tremendous laughter? What happened to Mahakashyap? In Buddhist scriptures, nothing is mentioned—only this solitary anecdote, that's all. When Buddha is gone, Mahakashyap is forgotten; then serious long-faces start organizing. Who will listen to the laughter? And Mahakashyap will recede back. Why bother?—these serious people are fighting so much that a man who loves laughing will get out of this mad mob of competitors: "Who is going to be the head of the Buddha *Sangha*, of the Order of Buddha?"—and politics enters, and fighting, and voting, and everything. Mahakashyap is simply lost. Where did he die?—nobody knows. Nobody knows the real heir of Buddha. Many centuries, almost six centuries pass; then another man, Bodhidharma, reaches China. Again Mahakashyap's name is heard, because Bodhidharma says, "I'm not a follower of the organized Buddhist religion. I have received my message through a direct line of Masters. It started with Buddha giving a flower to Mahakashyap, and I am the sixth." Who were the other four in between?—but it became a secret thing. When mad people become too ambitious and politics becomes strong, laughter goes secret. It becomes a private, intimate relationship. Silently, Mahakashyap must have delivered his message to somebody, and then he to somebody else, and he to Bodhidharma.

Why did Bodhidharma go to China? Zen Buddhists have been asking for centuries, "Why? Why did this Bodhidharma go to China?" I know; there is a reason: the Chinese are more joyous people than Indians, more delighted with life and small things, more colorful. It must be the reason why Bodhidharma travelled so long, crossed the whole of the Himalayas to seek and search for people who could laugh with him, and who were not serious, not great scholars and philosophers, and this and that. No, China has not created great philosophers like India has. It has created a few great mystics like Lao Tzu and Chuang Tzu, but they all are laughing Buddhas. It must be that Bodhidharma's search towards China was a search for people who were non-serious, light.

My whole effort here is to make you light, non-serious, laughing. People come to me, particularly Indians, to complain that: "What type of sannyasins are you creating? They don't look like sannyasins. A sannyasin has to be a serious person, almost dead, a corpse. These people laugh and dance and hug each other. This is

unbelievable! Sannyasins doing this?" And I tell them, "Who else?
Who else can do that?—only sannyasins can laugh."
So Vidya, very good—laugh, enjoy, be more and more light.

The third question:

> Every lecture is to be an injection of life. At times I go out
> permeated by your presence, at times confused; anyhow, rich,
> new. I feel loving and loved by life. Instead, after even the
> sweetest darshan, I feel deeply frustrated. Could you say
> something about this?

The question is from Prapatti.
Yes, I know this happens. This has to happen. It is with a deep
consideration; I want it to happen that way. When you are listening
to me in the morning talk, I'm not talking to you personally. I'm
not talking to anybody personally. I'm not talking to anybody in
particular, I'm simply talking. Of course, you are not involved in it,
you are just a listener. Even if I hit you on your heads you can
always think it is for others, you can always find excuses: "Bhagwan is doing it to others, doing well." You can always exclude
yourself.
But when you come to *darshan* in the evening, I am talking to
you in particular, Prapatti. Then I hit you and you cannot avoid it.
And I know you need many shocks, because there is no other way to
wake you. The alarm has to be jarring and hard, and when you
would like to sleep, the alarm disturbs you. In fact, exactly in those
moments when you would have really liked to sleep, suddenly the
alarm goes.
Whenever I see any fragment of sleep travelling in your mind, I
have to hit you hard. And of course, in darshan you are facing me;
it is an encounter, and you feel frustrated. If you understand you
will feel fulfilled, not frustrated. If you understand you will see why
I hit you so hard. I am not your enemy. It must be out of compassion that I hit you so hard. If you understand me, you will feel
grateful that I bother to hit you. Let me tell you a few anecdotes.
A man went into a large store and bought some groceries. As he
was waiting for his change, he kicked the assistant in the leg. Then
he apologized: "I'm awfully sorry, sir. It is a nervous thing I have."

"Why don't you see a doctor about it then?" the assistant asked him.

Soon he returned to the store. This time, nothing happened at all.

"I see you are cured," said the assistant. "Did you see the psychiatrist?"

"I did," said the man.

"How did he cure you?" the assistant asked.

"Well," said the man, "when I kicked him in the leg, he kicked me back—and very hard."

So when you come to me, remember: if you kick me, I am going to kick you very hard. And sometimes even when you don't kick, I kick. Your ego has to be shattered; that's why the frustration. The frustration is of the ego, it is not yours. I don't allow your ego. I don't give any visible or invisible support to it. But in the morning talks, it is very easy. Whatsoever hammering I do is for others, and whatsoever you feel good with is for you; you can choose. But not so in the evening.

Let me tell you another anecdote.

She: "Do you love me with all your heart and soul?"

He: "Uh huh."

She: "Do you think I am the most beautiful girl in the world, bar none?"

He: "Yeah."

She: "Do you think my lips are like rose petals, my eyes limpid pools, my hair like silk?"

He: "Yup."

She: "Oh, you say the nicest things."

In the morning talk, it is very easy; you can believe whatsoever you want to believe I am saying to you. But in the evening darshan, it is impossible.

But remember that I hit you hard to help you. It is out of compassion and love. When a stranger comes to me, I don't hit him, even in darshan. In fact, I don't make any contact, because all contact from me is going to be like an electric shock. Only with sannyasins am I hard, and I am harder when I see that your potentiality is greater. Prapatti has a great potential. She can grow and flower beautifully, and in no time, but she needs great pruning. It hurts. Remember, whenever it hurts, always watch . . . and you will see it is the ego that feels hurt, not you. Dropping the ego, chopping the ego, one day you will arise out of it, beyond the clouds. And then you will understand my compassion and my love, not before it.

ters for their whole lives; nothing is wrong. If you remain true to love, it

People ask me, "Won't you help us if we are not sannyasins?" I'm ready to help, but it will be difficult for you. Once you are a sannyasin, you become part of me. Then I can do whatsoever I like to do, and I don't bother even to ask your permission; there is no need. Once you have become a sannyasin, you have given me all permission, you have given me all authority. When you take sannyas you are giving a gesture to me, showing your heart. You are saying, "Now, I am here. Do whatsoever you like." And of course, I have to cut many parts which have become wrongly joined in you. It is going to be almost a surgery. Many things have to be removed, undone. Many new things have to be added to you. Your energy has to be re-channelized; it is moving in wrong directions. So it is going to be almost a dismantling, and then a re-creation. It is going to be almost a chaos. But remember always, only out of chaos are dancing stars born; there is no other way.

The last question:

In the East, it has been stressed that one should stay with a person, one person, in a love relationship. In the West, now people float from one relationship to another. Which are you in favor of?

I am in favor of love.

Let me explain it to you: be true to love, and don't bother about partners. Whether one partner or many partners is not the question. The question is whether you are true to love. If you live with a woman or with a man and you don't love him, you live in sin. If you are married to somebody and you don't love that person and you still go on living with him, making love to him or her, you are committing a sin against love . . . and love is God.

You are deciding against love for social comforts, conveniences, formalities. It is as wrong as if you go and rape a woman you don't love. You go and rape a woman; it is a crime—because you don't love the woman and the woman does not love you. But the same happens if you live with a woman and you don't love her. Then it is a rape—socially accepted, of course, but it is a rape—and you are going against the God of love.

So, like in the East, people have decided to live with one partner for their whole lives; nothing is wrong. If you remain true to love, it is one of the most beautiful things to remain with one person, because intimacy grows. But, ninety-nine per cent are the possibilities that there is no love; you only live together. And by living together a certain relationship grows which is only of living together, not of love. And don't mistake it for love. But if it is possible, if you love a person and live the whole life with him or with her, a great intimacy will grow and love will have deeper and deeper revelations to make to you. It is not possible if you go on changing partners very often. It is as if you go on changing a tree from one place to another, then another; then it never grows roots anywhere. To grow roots, a tree needs to remain in one place. Then it goes deeper; then it becomes stronger. Intimacy is good, and to remain in one commitment is beautiful, but the basic necessity is love. If a tree is rooted in a place where there are only rocks and they are killing the tree, then it is better to remove it. Then don't insist that it should remain in the one place. Remain true to life—remove the tree, because now it is going against life.

In the West, people are changing—too many relationships. Love is killed in both ways. In the East it is killed because people are afraid to change; in the West it is killed because people are afraid to remain with one partner for a longer time—afraid because it becomes a commitment. So before it becomes a commitment, change. So you remain floating and free, so a certain licentiousness is growing. And in the name of freedom, love is almost crushed, starved to death. Love has suffered both ways: in the East people cling to security, comfort, formality; in the West they cling to their ego's freedom, non-commitment—but love is suffering both ways.

I am in favor of love. I am neither Eastern nor Western, and I don't bother to which society you belong. I belong to no society. I am in favor of love. Always remember: if it is a love relationship, good.

While love lasts remain in it, and remain in it as deeply committed as possible. Remain in it as totally as possible; be absorbed by the relationship. Then love will be able to transform you. But if there is no love, it is better to change. But then, don't become an addict of change. Don't make it a habit. Don't let it become a mechanical habit that you have to change after each two or three years as one has to change one's car after each two or three years, or after each year. A new model comes, so what to do?—you have to change your car. Suddenly, you come across a new woman. It is not much different. A woman is a woman, as a man is a man. The differences are only secondary because it is a question of energy. The female energy is female energy. In each woman all women are

represented, and in each man all men are represented. The differences are very superficial: the nose is a little longer, or it is not a
little longer; the hair is blond or brunette—small differences, just
on the surface. Deep down, the question is of female and male
energy. So if love is there, stick to it. Give it a chance to grow. But
if it is not there, change before you become addicted to a relationship without love.

A young wife in the confessional box asked the priest about
contraceptives. "You must not use them," said the priest. "They are
against God's law. Take a glass of water."

"Before, or after?" asked the wife.

"Instead!" replied the priest.

You ask me whether to follow the Eastern way or the Western
way. Neither; you follow the divine way. And what is the divine
way?—remain true to love. If love is there, everything is permitted.
If love is not there, nothing is permitted. If you don't love your wife
don't touch her, because that is trespassing. If you don't love a
woman, don't sleep with her; that is going against the law of love,
and that is the ultimate law. Only when you love is everything
permitted.

Somebody asked Augustine of Hippo, "I am a very uneducated
man and I cannot read scriptures and great theology books. You
just give me a small message. I'm very foolish and my memory is
also not good, so you just give me a gist, so I can remember it and
follow it." Augustine was a great philosopher, a great saint, and he
had delivered great sermons, but nobody had asked for just a gist.
He closed his eyes, he meditated for hours, it is said. And the man
said, "Please, if you have found, just tell me so I can go, because I
have been waiting for hours." Augustine said, "I cannot find anything else except this: love, and everything else is permitted to you.
Just love."

Jesus says, "God is love." I would like to say to you, love is God.
Forget all about God; love will do. Remain courageous enough to
move with love; no other consideration should be made. If you
consider love, everything will become possible to you.

First, don't move with a woman or man you don't love. Don't
move just out of whim; don't move just out of lust. Find out
whether the desire to be committed to a person has arisen in you.
Are you ripe enough to make a deep contact? Because that contact
is going to change your whole life. And when you make the contact,
make it so truthfully. Don't hide from your beloved or your
lover—be true. Drop all false faces that you have learned to wear.

Drop all masks. Be true. Reveal your whole heart; be nude. Between two lovers there should not be any secrets, otherwise love is not. Drop all secrecy. It is politics; secrecy is politics. It should not be in love. You should not hide anything. Whatsoever arises in your heart should remain transparent to your beloved, and whatsoever arises in her heart should remain transparent to you. You should become two transparent beings to each other. By and by, you will see that through each other you are growing to a higher unity.

By meeting the woman outside, by really meeting, loving her, committing yourself to her being, dissolving into her, melting into her, you will, by and by, start meeting the woman that is within you; you will start meeting the man that is within you. The outer woman is just a path to the inner woman; and the outer man is also just a path to the inner man. The real orgasm happens inside you when your inner man and woman meet. That is the meaning of the Hindu symbolism of *ardhanarishwar*. You must have seen Shiva: half man, half woman. Each man is half man, half woman; each woman is half woman, half man. It has to be so, because half of your being comes from your father and half of your being comes from your mother. You are both. An inner orgasm, an inner meeting, an inner union is needed. But to reach to that inner union you will have to find a woman outside who responds to the inner woman, who vibrates your inner being, and your inner woman which is lying fast asleep, awakes. Through the outer woman, you have to meet the inner woman; and the same for the man.

So if the relationship continues for a long period, it will be better, because that inner woman needs time to be awakened. As it is happening in the West—hit-and-run affairs—the inner woman has no time, the inner man has no time to rise and become awake. By the time there is a stirring, the woman is gone ... another woman, with another vibration, with another vibe. And of course, if you go on changing your woman and your man you will become neurotic, because so many things, so many sounds will enter into your being, and so many different qualities of vibrations that you will be at a loss to find your inner woman. It will be difficult. And the possibility is that you may become an addict to change. You will just start enjoying change. Then you are lost.

The outer woman is just a way to the inner woman, and the outer man is the way to the inner man. And the ultimate yoga, the ultimate *unio mystica* happens inside you. And when that happens, then you are free of all women and all men. Then you are free of man and womanhood. Then suddenly, you go beyond; then you are neither.

This is what transcendence is. This is what *brahmacharya* is. Then you attain again to your pure virginity; your original nature is again claimed. In Patanjali's terminology, it is *kaivalya*.

BOOKS BY BHAGWAN SHREE RAJNEESH

THE ULTIMATE ALCHEMY VOLS I AND II
(discourses on the Atma Pooja Upanishad)

THE BOOK OF THE SECRETS VOLS I—V
(discourses on Tantra)

THE SUPREME DOCTRINE
(discourses on the Kenopanishad)

VEDANTA: SEVEN STEPS TO SAMADHI
(discourses on the Akshya Upanishad)

YOGA: THE ALPHA AND THE OMEGA VOLS I— X
(discourses on Patanjali's Yoga Sutras)

MY WAY: THE WAY OF THE WHITE CLOUDS
(talks based on questions)

ROOTS AND WINGS
(talks based on questions)

THE EMPTY BOAT
(discourses on Chuang Tzu)

NO WATER, NO MOON
(discourses on Zen)

THE MUSTARD SEED
(discourses on the sayings of Jesus)

WHEN THE SHOE FITS
(discourses on Chuang Tzu)

NEITHER THIS NOR THAT
(discourses on Sosan—Zen)

... AND THE FLOWERS SHOWERED
(discourses on Zen)

RETURNING TO THE SOURCE
(discourses on Zen)

THE HIDDEN HARMONY
(discourses on the fragments of Heraclitus)

TANTRA: THE SUPREME UNDERSTANDING
(discourses on Tilopa's Song of Mahamudra)

THE GRASS GROWS BY ITSELF
(discourses on Zen stories)

UNTIL YOU DIE
(discourses on the Sufi Way)

JUST LIKE THAT
(discourses on Sufi stories)

TAO: THE THREE TREASURES VOLS I—IV
(discourses on Lao Tzu)

THE TRUE SAGE
(discourses on Hassidic stories)

NIRVANA: THE LAST NIGHTMARE
(discourses on Zen stories)

HAMMER ON THE ROCK
(a darshan diary I)

ABOVE ALL, DON'T WOBBLE
(darshan diary II)

NOTHING TO LOSE BUT YOUR HEAD
(darshan diary III)

THE SEARCH
(discourses on the ten Zen Bulls)

COME FOLLOW ME VOLS I—IV
(discourses on the life of Jesus)

ANCIENT MUSIC IN THE PINES
(discourses on Zen)

DANG DANG DOKO DANG
(discourses on Zen)

THE BELOVED VOLS I AND II
(discourses on the Baul Mystics)

A SUDDEN CLASH OF THUNDER
(discourses on Zen)

THE DISCIPLINE OF TRANSCENDENCE VOL I
(discourses on the sayings of Buddha)

THE ART OF DYING
(discourses on Hassidic stories)

ECSTASY: THE FORGOTTEN LANGUAGE
(discourses on the songs of Kabir)

BE REALISTIC: PLAN FOR A MIRACLE
(darshan diary IV)

GET OUT OF YOUR OWN WAY
(darshan diary V)

foreign editions

THE BOOK OF THE SECRETS VOL I
(Harper and Row, USA)

THE BOOK OF THE SECRETS VOL I
(Thames and Hudson, UK)

NO WATER NO MOON
(Sheldon Press, UK)

STRAIGHT TO FREEDOM
(Indian edition: UNTIL YOU DIE)
(Sheldon Press, UK)

ONLY ONE SKY
(Indian edition: TANTRA: THE SUPREME

UNDERSTANDING)
(Dutton, USA)

I AM THE GATE
(Harper and Row, USA)

MEDITATION: THE ART OF ECSTASY
(Harper and Row, USA)

TANTRA, SPIRITUALITY AND SEX
(Rainbow Bridge, USA)

THE MUSTARD SEED
(Sheldon Press, UK)

TANTRA: THE SUPREME UNDERSTANDING
(Sheldon Press, UK)

NEITHER THIS NOR THAT
(Sheldon Press, UK)

DIMENSIONS BEYOND THE KNOWN
(Sheldon Press, UK)

THE PSYCHOLOGY OF THE ESOTERIC
(Harper and Row, USA)

WHEN THE SHOE FITS
(DeVorss and Co, USA)

THE GRASS GROWS BY ITSELF
(DeVorss and Co, USA)

THE MUSTARD SEED
(Harper and Row, USA)

translations

TANTRA: SONZAI NO UTA
(Japanese—Merkmal Ltd, Tokyo)

TANTRA: HET ALLERHOOGSTE INZICHT
(Dutch—Ankh-Hermes)

MEDITAZIONE DINAMICA
(Italian—Edizioni Mediterranee, Rome)

YO SOY LA PUERTA
(Spanish—Editorial Diana S.A., Mexico)

LE LIVRE DES SECRETS VOL I
(French—Les Editions A.T.P. Paris)

LA RIVOLUZIONE INTERIORE
(Italian—Armenia Editore)

HU MEDITATION OG KOSMIC ORGASME
(Danish—Borgens Forlag A/S)

Il LIBRO DEI SEGRETI VOL I
(Italian—Armenia Editore)

KYUKYOKU NO TABI
(Japanese—Merkmal Ltd, Tokyo)

DE WEG VAN DE WITTE WOLKEN
(Dutch—Arcanum)

HET ZOEKEN
(Dutch—Ankh-Hermes)

MEDITATIE, DE KUNST VAN DE EXTASE
(Dutch—Ankh-Hermes)

HAMMERE DEN FELSEN
(German—Fischer Taschenbuch Verlag)

RAJNEESH MEDITATION CENTERS

INDIA

SHREE RAJNEESH ASHRAM, 17 Koregaon Park, Poona 411 001
Tel: 28127

SAGAR DEEP, 52 Ridge Road, Malabar Hill, Bombay 400 006
Tel: 364783

USA

ANANDA, 29 East 28th Street, New York, N.Y. 10016
Tel: 212 686 3261

DHYANTARU, 375a Huron Ave, Cambridge, Mass. 02138
Tel: 617 491 2671

BODHITARU, 7231 SW 62nd Place, Miami, Florida 33143

MAITREYA, 431 W 20th St, New York, N.Y. 10011
Tel: 212 924 2069

SARVAM, 6412 Luzon Ave., Washington D.C. 20012
Tel: 202 726 1712

GEETAM, Box 576, Highway 18, Lucerne Valley, California 92356
Tel: 714 248 6163

PARAS, 4301 24th Street, San Francisco, California 94114

DEVALAYAM, P.O. Box 592, G.P.O. Kansas City, Missouri 69141

PREMSAGAR, P.O. Box 2862, Chapel Hill, North Carolina 27514

CANADA

ARVIND, 1330 Renfrew St, Vancouver, B.C.

ENGLAND

KALPTARU, Top Floor, 10a Belmont St, London NW1
Postal address: 28 Oak Village, London NW 5 4QN
Tel: 01 267 8304

NIRVANA, 82 Bell Street, London NW1 Tel: 01 262 0991

PREMTARU, Church Farm House, Field Dalling, Holt, Norfolk

SURYODAYA, The Old Rectory, Gislingham, by Diss, Nr. Eye, Suffolk

TUSHITA, North Moreton, Didcot, Oxfordshire 119BA

ANURODHA, Flat I, 30 Church Road, Moseley, Birmingham 15

SCOTLAND
GOURISHANKAR, 9 Ravensdean Gardens, Penicuik, Midlothian
Tel: Penicuik 73034
PRASTHAN, 21 Wilmot Road, Glasgow C13 1XL

FRANCE
PREMPATH, 45-390 Desmonts
SHANTIDWEEP, 25 Avenue Pierre Premier de Serbie, Paris XVIe
Tel: 720   7930

SPAIN
PALASH, Can Bonet, Sta. Gertrudis, Ibiza, Baleares

HOLLAND
AMITABH, Pieter Paauwstr 6 , Amsterdam

DENMARK
ANAND NIKETAN, Skindergade 3, DK—1159, Copenhagen K
Tel: 01   11   79   09

ITALY
ARIHANT, Via Cacciatori delle Alpi 19, 20019 Settimo Milanese,
Milan

SWITZERLAND
SATYAM, Schilberg, 16 Rue Richemont, 1202, Geneva

WEST GERMANY
PURVODAYA, D-8051 Margaretenried, Fongi-Hof Tel: 08764   426
SHREYAS,8 Munich 60, Raucheneggerstr. 4/11
ANANDLOK, 1 Berlin 61, Mehringdamm 61
Postal address: 1 Berlin 61, Luckenwalderstr. 11

JAPAN
ASHEESH, 5-4-17 Kichijoji-Kitamachi, Musashino-shi, Tokyo
Tel: 0422   53   6483

EAST AFRICA
ANAND NEED, P.O. Box 72424, Nairobi, Kenya

SOUTH AFRICA
BODHISATTVA, P.O. Box 1, New Germany, Natal

BRAZIL
PURNAM, Caixa Postale 1946, Porto Alegre, Rio G. do Sul
Tel: 425588
SOMA, Rua Caraibas 1179, Casa 9, 05020 Pompeia, Sao Paulo

AUSTRALIA
SHANTI SADAN, Havelock Clinic, 1 Havelock St, West Perth,
Western Australia 6005
DEVAYAN, 25 Martyn St, Cairns, Queensland 4870

NEW ZEALAND
SHANTI NIKETAN, 9 Edenvale Road, Mount Eden, Auckland

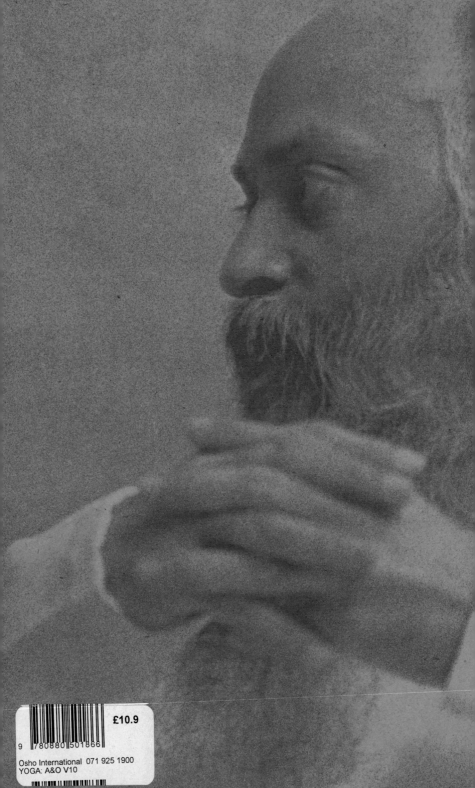

£10.9

9 780880 501866

Osho International 071 925 1900
YOGA: A&O V10